SECRETS OF
THE
GOLDEN
DOOR

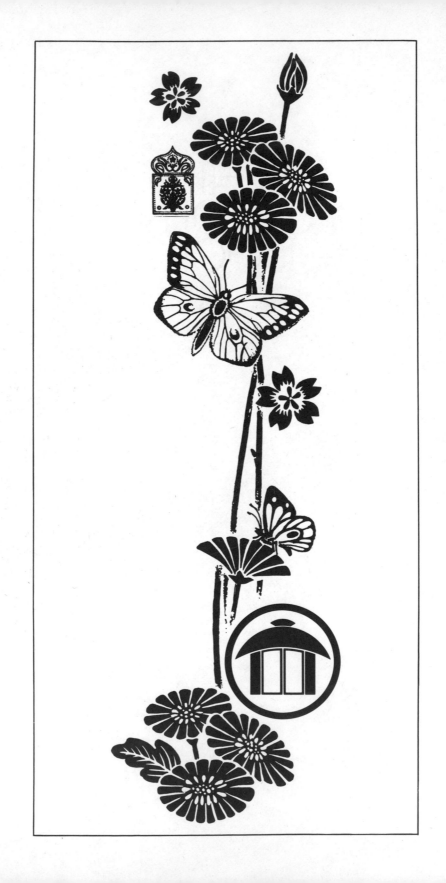

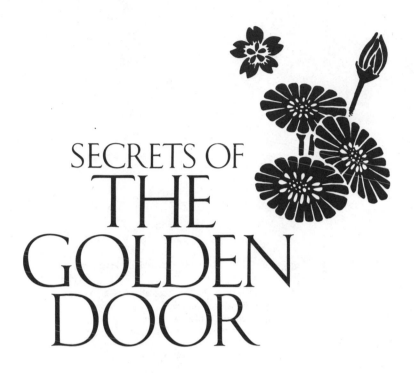

SECRETS OF
THE
GOLDEN
DOOR

DEBORAH SZEKELY
MAZZANTI

WILLIAM MORROW AND COMPANY, INC.
NEW YORK   1977

Printed in the United States of America.

2   3   4   5   6   7   8   9   10

Library of Congress Cataloging in Publication Data

Mazzanti, Deborah Szekely.
    Secrets of The Golden Door.

    1. Health. 2. Beauty, Personal. 3. Golden Door
(Health resort) I. Title.
RA776.5.M39   613   77-2722
ISBN 0-688-03237-0

BOOK DESIGN   CARL WEISS

DEDICATED to Edmond Bordeaux Szekely, teacher, philosopher, and impossible man, whom I met in 1933, married in 1939, and divorced in 1969; who gave me my life's work and my two children.

DEDICATED also to the 250,000 people who have crossed my threshold and who have taught me even as I taught them. Their trust inspired me to seek the answers reprinted within these pages.

AND WITH A SPECIAL WORD for both my children, Alex and Livia Szekely, and Vincent E. Mazzanti, my husband. Their love sustains me and their pride in me makes me do my very best.

ACKNOWLEDGMENTS

WITH GRATEFUL THANKS to Ned Riley, Livia Szekely, and John Poppy, who tidied my reams of untidy notes, and to Roberta Ridgely, who made it all so readable.

To Marge Newby Samuels, who has been the exercise choreographer at The Golden Door almost since the day we opened.

To Susanne Mitzkat, one of the most popular of our fitness specialists, who posed for the exercises in Chapter IV, and to Charles Schneider, who has been The Golden Door photographer since before we opened.

To Michel Strout, Ray Piper, and Jinx Morgan for their contributions to the menus and recipes in Chapter VII.

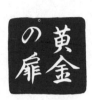 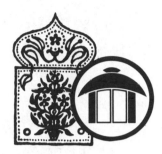

CONTENTS

Happiness is difficult to find within,

impossible to find elsewhere.

—SEBASTIEN CHAMFORT

(Copied from the flyleaf of *The Dictionary of Love,* given to me on my fourteenth birthday by Edmond Bordeaux Szekely.)

A NOTE FROM
THE AUTHOR

I feel I want to begin by telling you something about myself, because The Golden Door is such an intensely personal extension of me—of what I have learned in the rather unusual circumstances of my growing up and my adult life. This projection of my life's experiences into The Golden Door is what has made it unique among spas. In nearly forty years of caring for my guests, I have evolved a very activist philosophy. I apply it at The Golden Door. The result is a galvanizing difference in the later lives of almost every guest who visits there.

I SUPPOSE THE FIRST CHAPTER OF MY ADULT LIFE BEGAN IN 1940, WHEN my husband, Professor Edmond Bordeaux Szekely, and I (a bride just one month past eighteen) drove down a dusty corrugated road leading to an old Spanish land grant in Baja California, Mexico, called Rancho La Puerta ("Ranch of the Door"). We sat on silver plush upholstery in an only slightly dilapidated 1928 Cadillac with cut-crystal bud vases between its side windows; it towed a handmade, silver-painted trailer box which contained all our worldly goods.

13

There, at Rancho La Puerta, we pioneered the basic approach to exercising and eating that would later become famous. We did this by developing the Activity Day. Till then few had considered how to replace the missing ingredient in modern life that once was the pre-requisite for all living beings—continuous movement. To gather food, primitive man and animal alike were preoccupied with a dawn-to-dusk search. We translated this dawn-to-dusk migration into the Activity Day. And this is fundamental to the fantastic results that have made The Golden Door world-famous.

It is a weird feeling to be required to explain how you came upon an original approach. At one point many years ago I began by saying to myself, "Here we are in the age of enlightenment. Why then the lack of well-being? Is it that we are leading our lives as if our bodies didn't really exist? What would be the most sensible means of re-adjustment?"

That I should have asked such questions and looked for answers was not surprising in view of my experience. I had neither medical training nor degree. But I possessed a one-of-a-kind background in exploring theories of health and natural living.

I must have been four years old when my mother became a vice-president of the New York Vegetarian Society. That would make the year 1926. Besides being vegetarian, my family also was fruitarian—meaning we ate nothing but raw fruits, vegetables, and nuts.

Almost every weekend we hiked to a different health camp. Midweek I fell asleep listening to health lectures all over Manhattan.

When I was seven, in 1929, the impact of the Great Depression hit us —but differently than it hit most New Yorkers. There wasn't much for fruitarians to eat. Of course, we too were suddenly poor, and many fresh fruits and nuts became not only expensive, but simply unavailable. Faced with a choice between starvation or relinquishing their principles, my parents decided to spend what money was left on steamship tickets; and so we sailed to Tahiti.

When my parents placed me in a convent school before going off to assess the other islands, they didn't realize that no one there spoke English. The school's everyday language was Tahitian; its second official language was French. Somehow I got through my first day at the convent without mishap. I credit my successes since that time to my exceptional vitality and my ability to observe. I guess it all began at that school in Tahiti, because there I had to learn not by listening, but by watching.

It was while we were in Tahiti that we met Professor Edmond Bordeaux Szekely. He had spent his youth researching early civilizations and searching for ways to apply natural living to an increasingly unnatural culture. He became the strongest influence in the life of my family. When we left the South Pacific after four and a half years, we were determined to live only half of each year in a city, and to spend the other half in a primitive community.

We spent many summers in Professor Szekely's health camps. This took us from Lake Elsinore in southern California to Rio Corona in Tamaulipas, Mexico. I spent my teen-age years listening to the small but motley group (health tramps and peers of the realm, faddists and scholars) who then comprised the health enthusiasts of the world.

I graduated from high school in 1938, when I was just sixteen. My mother decided that I was too young for college. Instead, I followed my family to Central Mexico, where Professor Szekely had now set up a new health camp. Joining him, we learned that his secretary had just been called home to England by the death of his father. Since the Professor was totally helpless about day-to-day practical details, I pitched in to help and remained after my parents returned to California. I proved such an efficient secretary and aide that, when my parents wrote to say it was time for me to return home to resume my education, he married me. That was 1939; we were to remain married until 1969.

Back to 1940: Professor Szekely was concerned both about the impending expiration of his U. S. immigration visa and by whispered rumors concerning probable internment of aliens if America should be drawn into the Second World War. A captain in the Romanian reserves who was now a man without a country, he chose to emigrate to Mexico. A happy and obedient new wife, I accompanied him. Together, on June 6, 1940, we opened our first spa, Rancho La Puerta, in Tecate, Baja California. As I have said, this was when my adult life really began.

From the beginning we experimented. We read and discussed and tried every health discipline and diet theory you're hearing about now: bean sprouts and acidophilus milk, total fasting and interval fasting, the grape cure, the mucus-free diet, morning walks, and mud baths. I have

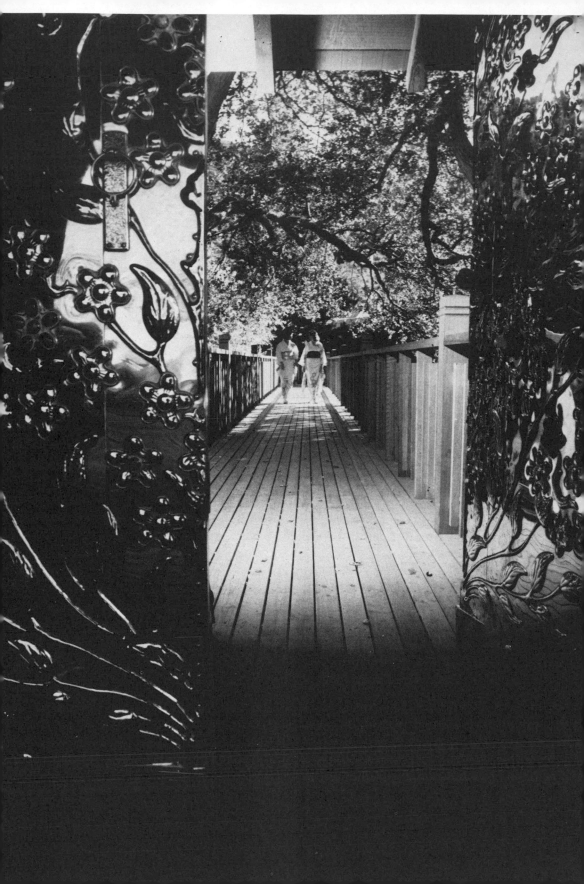

never come across anything that we didn't try once. Today every so-
called new diet plan or exercise idea is, to me, *déjà vu*. Direct observa-
tion is the key to everything I've learned.

Rancho La Puerta, The Golden Door's forerunner, grew and grew,
eventually expanding into the largest health resort of its kind. By now,
almost a quarter of a million guests have stepped through its welcoming
archway.

I celebrated our twentieth wedding anniversay by opening The
Golden Door, a resort planned from the start to be small, intimate, and
my version of heaven. We began with only twelve guests each week.
(Even today we remain the world's smallest major spa.) But after a time
our marriage began to falter, and in 1969 we were divorced.

Another milestone, my fiftieth birthday, marked the beginning of
Book II in my life. On that date—May 3, 1972—I became engaged to
Vincent E. Mazzanti, the wise and warm and wonderfully understanding
psychoanalyst whom I married in June. And in that same year I reached
the decision to build a new Golden Door; over thirty years of experience
and dreams were poured into an establishment which was to be hailed
as "the ultimate spa."

Today The Golden Door accepts just thirty guests at any one time,
so that our staff of eighty-seven can give the most meticulous attention
to each one. The location, in a beautiful little California valley, affords
both seclusion and year-round comfort. In such ideally protective surroundings one can dare to advance new ideas and concepts.

Most of our guests take out into the world heightened vitality—the
desire and ability to create something of a new self, to live more and
more in a world of his or her own choosing.

My dearest hope is that this is what will happen to you as you read
this book.

DEBORAH SZEKELY MAZZANTI

CHAPTER I

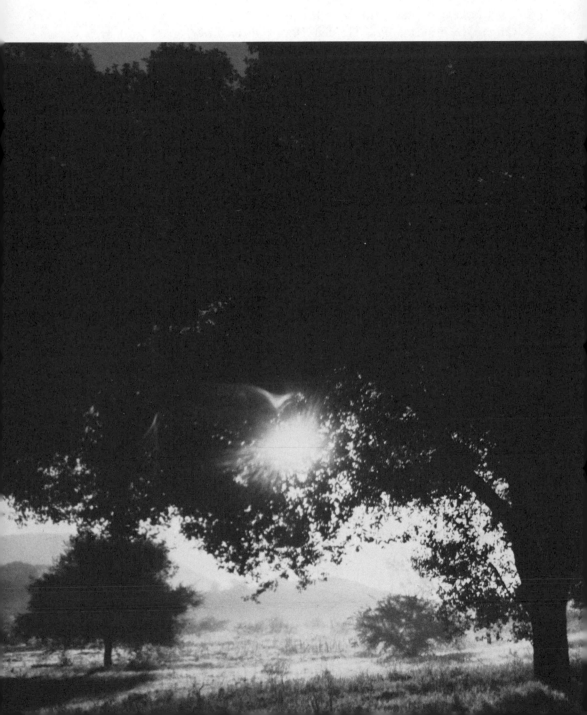

JOY,
THE SECRET
INGREDIENT

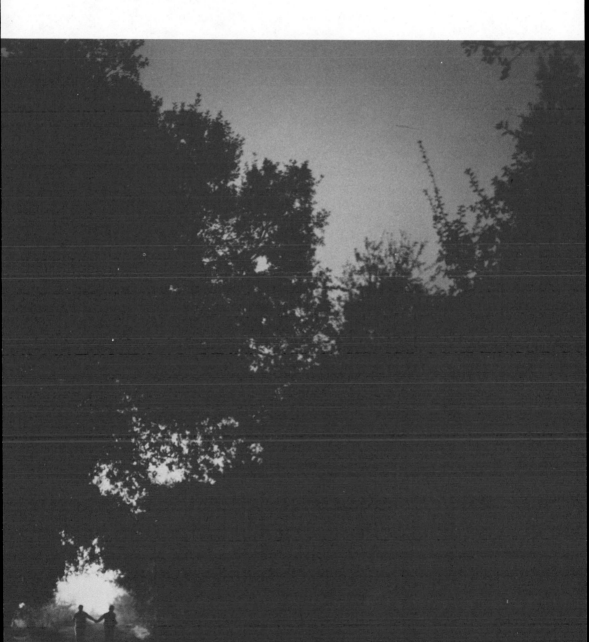

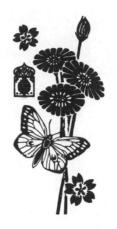

T HE PARAMOUNT PURPOSE OF THIS BOOK IS TO POINT YOU TOWARD joy—whether by talking about getting to know your body, or about cooking some of the most delicious food you've ever tasted. Joy is what our guests come seeking at The Golden Door, and it is what they take home. It's the secret I want you to make your own as you read these pages.

What I'm about to tell you is as much a matter of *context* for your life and its varying aspects as it is a matter of *content*. Absorb everything in your own time, in your own way, and in your own sequence. A valid program must accommodate itself to the swirling patterns of my guests' everyday lives after they are home again—and to *your* daily activities.

□ HEALTH TO GO

Years go by, names change, but people and their problems remain the same. The Golden Door program has been shared by such widely divergent personalities as Jean Arthur and Barbra Streisand; Dorothy

Kirsten and Roberta Flack; Bess Myerson and Shana Alexander; Jane Russell and Dyan Cannon; Barbara Howar and the late Judy Garland; the Gabors—mother Jolie and daughters Eva and Zsa Zsa; and the forever young and forever active such as Debbie Reynolds and Dinah Shore. During Men's Week, our notables have ranged from Burt Lancaster to William Holden; Bill Blass and Stanley Kramer to the late Aldous Huxley.

Those who return again and again, and seem to grow increasingly luminous with each visit, are the ones who have married their lives to a healthful year-round routine based on Golden Door guidelines.

There's nothing mysterious about developing habits that will stimulate you and give you verve. But you and the program you adopt for yourself must be characterized by balance rather than by overzealousness.

Trust me. At one extreme are depression, boredom, and fatigue; the Cookie Monster; obesity; and, eventually, alarming symptoms. At the opposite pole are Captain Bligh, nose to the grindstone, shoulder to the wheel, and *Achtung!* Aren't you relieved you'll be asked only to effect an appropriate balance between them? *Le juste milieu* is what the French call it, the point between two extremes—another name for The Golden Mean, another name for keeping things in a healthy perspective, another name for The Golden Door.

As The Golden Door philosophy is revealed to you, you'll recognize the profound relationship of your body and spirit. For many, this new relationship may be like a trip to a foreign land. When you begin such a trip you bring along a simple vocabulary, maps, and guidebooks. And these are what I hope to supply you with in this book—my secrets of The Golden Door. I am going to help you learn to listen and look intently—and to remember that your own reflection in the mirror is just the outer image of what is going on within.

With these thoughts in mind, you can begin your day at home just as we do at The Golden Door. Begin at the beginning, while still in bed and not really quite awake. Take a moment to feel your body. Count your toes and fingers just as you would a newborn baby's. (All there?) Here's where your mind/body are. This is your home, where *you* really live.

Now introduce your body to the day. First, two minutes of stretching and moving exercises, nude. Exercise before a full-length mirror, with your eyes wide open. Start at the top; stretch and embrace the world. Feel your freedom, breathe deeply, be aware that the air is touching you, wiggle your toes and identify the movement of each one. This feeling of wholeness, this sense of the mind/body in which you live with your inner and outer self, is what you are going to use to create your day and your entire life.

Hop quickly on the scales, for in planning your day you need to know whether yesterday built up your fuel reserves or depleted them.

Now, instead of your robe, put on your jogging suit. This is your commitment to yourself. If you are one of the lucky few who can exercise before breakfast, that's ideal. If you're a houseperson you may have to wait till the kids are off to school and everyone has left. If you work, you will have to set your alarm thirty minutes earlier. Believe me when I say a half-hour spent in exercise does far more for you than a half-hour passed in sleep.

It's your exercise routine that will get your day off to its real start. The important thing about exercise is that it becomes a daily habit, as much a reflex as breathing. You establish that by picking a time slot, a permanent one about which you never have to make any day-to-day decisions. After all, you weren't born with a toothbrush in your mouth; yet you brush your teeth at least twice a day without thinking. The kind of exercise you choose and the length of the exercise period are dealt with later in this book. Now I'm merely talking about the concept—the creation of a reflex, your own re-education.

Schedule your morning exercise program for Monday through Friday. Your Saturday and Sunday schedule can be fitted into your weekend plans. Exercise in the morning has many physiological and psychological benefits. Perhaps it has something to do with the rising of the sun, the singing of the birds, the lifting of the mist, and even the tug of the tides. There's a great uplift in the morning, gathering one's strengths, marshaling one's energies—all combining to help you enter your day with a strong feeling that you surround the day's tasks rather than the other way around.

For me the greatest benefit of morning exercise is the return home from the park, the feeling that God's in His heaven and all's right with the world. You will feel energized because you have set a goal and then achieved it with ease. This confidence will carry over into everything you do. I believe it's no coincidence that my friends who walk and jog and exercise invariably are the people of greatest achievement.

Just as you use exercise to get yourself up in the morning, also use it to wind down at night. There once was a time called twilight, the prelude for what many people feel is the most rewarding time of day—the evening. The work required for daily life was then completed, and people could live a little for themselves; we must recreate that bridge between the day's activities and the night's different pace.

When you arrive home, instead of turning on the TV set or making a drink, put on your jogging shoes, run around the block for ten minutes, or swim, or hop onto your Exercycle, or just go into the back bedroom and jump rope. It's not important what you do; the important thing is to change the pattern of tension and the pattern of breathing. But I will get to all this later. For now, remember your two exercise periods, one at the beginning of the day and one at the beginning of the evening.

Back to your breakfast. At the table, plan your day—not only its activities but the fuel necessary to power those activities. Look at your breakfast plate and think of the food before you as so much energy. This serving represents tennis, this the exercise you did this morning, and this, the hours you'll be seated at your desk.

Keep an accurate calendar of your day. Mark your lunch plans— whether you're having lunch out or just a cup of yogurt at your desk— and at the same time think about dinner. If you're a twosome both of you consider not only this evening's dinner but what your social schedule for the week will be. A big meal on Wednesday means a small meal on Thursday. Plan your meals with the same perspective as you do your other activities.

Breakfast in itself is simple. You'll find out all about that in the nutrition chapter and in the recipes that follow (pages 170–281).

For lunch, have two courses—an appetite-spoiler and lunch. Your appetite-spoiler should be eaten thirty minutes before your meal, either at home or at your desk before you leave for the restaurant. Its purpose is to lift your blood sugar (again, I'll amplify later). Then, for the restaurant eater, choose your lunch from the appetizers, the hors d'oeuvres, where you can control the portion. At home eat any low-calorie lunch.

Dinner is the principal meal—the main event. There are many tricks

to making the ritual of dinner psychologically and physiologically satisfying; you will learn about them later. But beware of the notion of
portion control, which restaurant owners base on how many calories it
will take to feed a large man. Cruise ship eating is based on enough
calories to power a man six feet, eight inches tall who weighs two hundred sixty pounds. I don't know your size, but I suspect it's a lot smaller
than that! If you went on such a cruise ship and stayed long enough you
probably would never measure that man's height, but you might approach his weight.

I'm going to help you find the way to put the right amount of food on
your plate in the first place, so that, after your meal, you will not feel
that you've denied yourself anything. I cannot give you X-ray vision so
that when you look at a dish you see the total calories. But I will tell
you how you can come close to this. And I will provide you with a
workable, companionable sort of guide so that you'll know when it's a
day to be very, very good; or when the day's been rough and it's o.k. to
eat a little more and soothe your ruffled feathers.

From infancy on people have developed the habit of cry, food, cry,
food. The baby cries. The mother soothes and feeds. Today, whenever
you're unhappy, it makes perfect sense that you should want to eat, to
unwind, to relax, to be stroked. This is not a habit you are going to
lose, but you'll learn how to make capital of it by seeing that everything
you do eat gives you maximum psychological and physiological pleasure.
Only then will you find genuine satisfaction without guilt—and with a
new awareness.

This awareness will lead you to selecting and choosing quality food
because a life of high vitality needs a high-octane fuel. Our Saturday-
go-to-the-supermarket shopping style is a direct descendant of those
Saturdays when people hitched up the buckboard and went into town
to do the marketing, to trade the surplus eggs for flour, and to buy the
oil and the sugar and the few other basics not grown at home. But in
those days food was fresh and unprocessed, whereas now what you buy
in your once-a-week shopping trip is processed—with most of the good
removed from it. The simpler the food, the better we do.

I'm going to teach you about those foods that give you maximum
energy with minimum effort. Freshness of course is an essential. Go to
your local market on Mondays and Wednesdays and Fridays, or when-

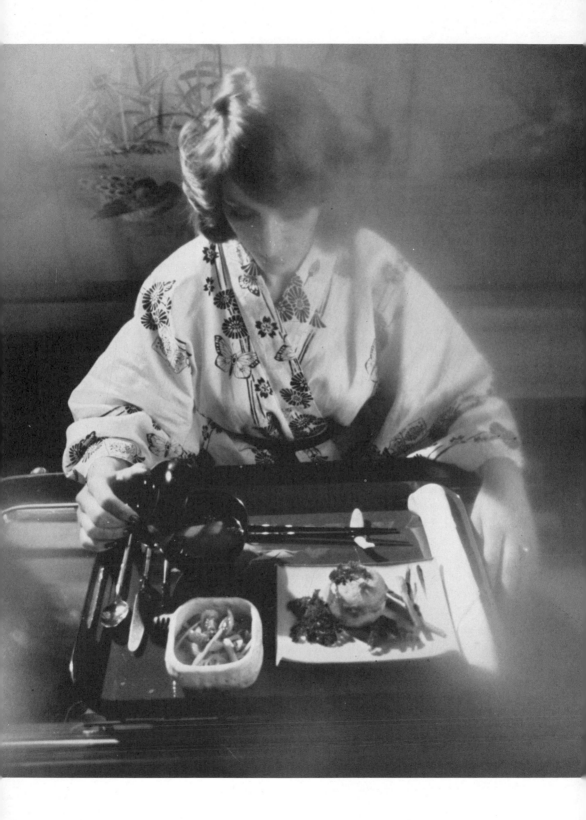

ever the market gets in its fresh produce. Dine on what is freshest and best that day, not what you read about in some diet plan or other.

Buy just the appropriate amount for the precise number of people you will be feeding in your household. With your daily calendar in your hand, marked with the meals eaten in and the meals out, you no longer will emerge from the supermarket with the overload carried out by so many people who needlessly are weighing down their mind/body and their life.

One of the most pleasing secrets I can pass on to you is that it takes one-third or one-fourth less time to prepare food when you're cooking for the actual needs of your own life—and not for leftovers or the refrigerator or the garbage disposal. If you require four carrots, cook four, not eight. If you're baking potatoes, think about the people who will be eating them: for this family member a small potato, for that one a larger potato. You'll begin to understand that we should eat according to the size we are and want to become. At all times the appropriate amount is very apparent.

The returning Golden Door guest (with rare exceptions, each and every guest returns) comes for the renewing and recharging that are part of a week devoted to listening to one's self. It's wonderfully gratifying for me to hear these guests talk. These are people who have resolved their onetime dilemma about how and when to exercise, how and what to eat. And they know all about the why. Now they are discovering with the greatest joy new dimensions to their mind/body connection. They have chosen to become drivers in their lives rather than passengers. You can choose too.

◻ AN INVITATION TO THE GOOD LIFE

Now, open your Golden Door. Begin.

Be practical. Don't bind yourself to a do-or-die approach. When you set yourself a modest goal at first, and reach it, and then set a more difficult one and reach that too, you're in training for success.

The essential Golden Door experiences involve these four parts of life and the proper balance between them all:

1. Movement

2. Relaxation
3. Nutrition
4. Joy

1. MOVEMENT is the touchstone of health. Ancient man moved from dawn till dusk. We still have need for daily, extensive, variegated exercise. The unextended body is the unlived-in body, the unlived-in life.

2. RELAXATION, at the opposite end of the spectrum, is no less important. A healthy body cannot be chronically contracted, pent-up, and pinched. It must be shown how to stretch and relax and how to know the joy of being still. One can have proper relaxation only when it has been preceded by vigorous physical movement.

3. NUTRITION is an elementary need. It truly is our fuel for both physical well-being and emotional health. Calories count—but far more important is the satisfaction your food gives you. A diet that deprives you of the pleasures of food cheats you of a valuable, even critical, part of your life. You are the sum total of what you eat.

4. JOY is the invisible and irreplaceable ingredient of true health. I don't need to remind you again that without the fusion of body and spirit, beauty cannot exist. If you approach the previous three essentials as obligations, you might conceivably build yourself a magnificent body. On the other hand, if you approach them joyfully as opportunities for self-enrichment, you can become wholly fit, fully adjusted to your environment, and ready for anything.

This psychological dimension of health is still mysterious and unpredictable. But it is never out of reach. And I believe that by eating sparingly of simple, wholesome, fresh, fresh foods, and by exercising creatively and relaxing deeply, we can enhance our inner peace.

□ GOOD HEALTH
IS YOUR BIRTHRIGHT

Don't sell yourself short as you make your future projections. Good health is not a privilege reserved for a few. To achieve it you merely need to reactivate an option you've held all along but haven't been *exercising*. Achieving a level of vibrant fitness is mostly a matter of letting your body enjoy itself.

And that also explains why this is not a diet book. In fact, it's an

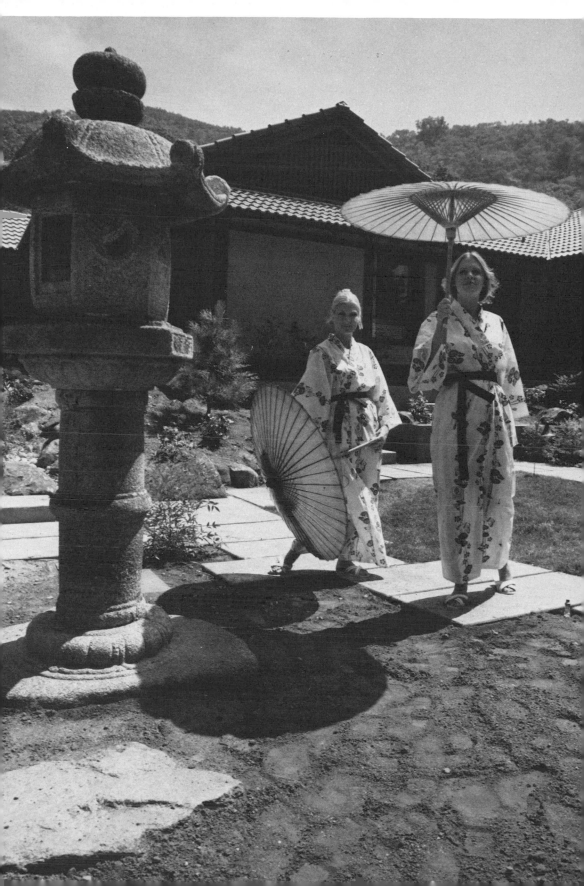

anti-diet book. The first three letters of the word "diet" tell the story all too well. To most people diets are a form of emotional suicide.

□ *ENJOY . . . ENJOY . . .*

Most health regimens fail because they lack the element of enjoyment. They cause a little flurry and then burn out their converts, some with food deprivation, others with boring calisthenics, and all with overwhelming invitations to guilt. Astoundingly, they ignore the principle that only your increasingly robust enjoyment of life—not a weight chart, not a gym routine, not an improved pulse rate—can keep you going.

That is why The Golden Door approach has nothing to do with food deprivation, calisthenics, or guilt. Guilt makes you unsatisfied and therefore hungry. Food is both a pleasure and a friend, and I mean to help you preserve that friendship; exercise can be dull, therefore I must help make it irresistible.

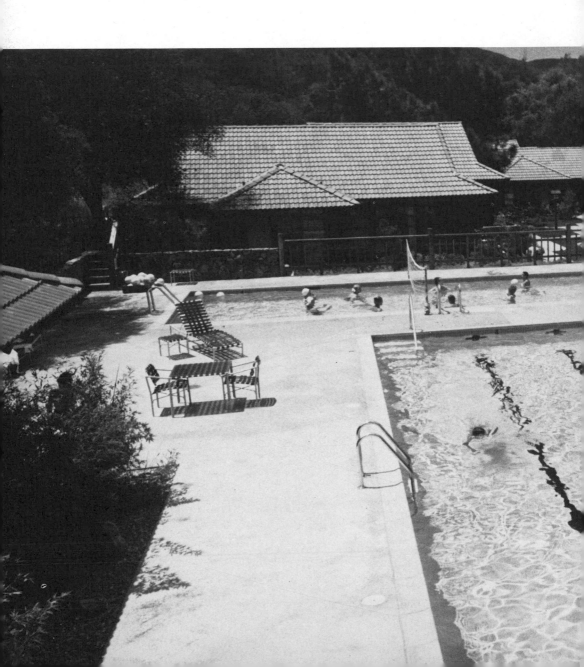

CHAPTER II

MOVEMENT:
THE DELIGHTS
OF PHYSICAL
ACTIVITY

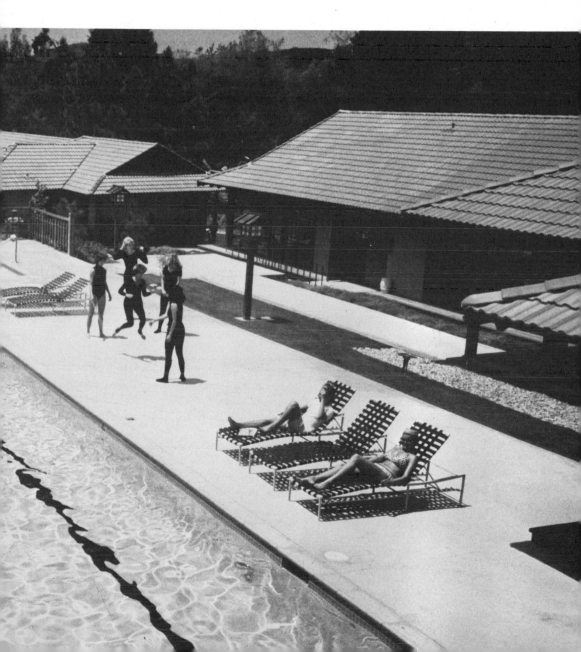

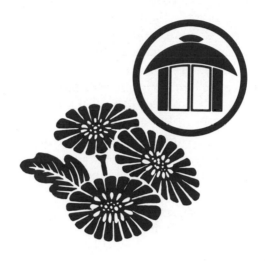

I F YOU WERE TO WRITE DOWN ALL OF YOUR PHYSICAL ACTIVITIES EVERY
day for a week, I could guess your age. Everybody has a perceptible
movement pattern, and most people over twenty-five are movement-
starved.

Age is nearly always signaled by decreasing circles of movement.
A young person moves in ever-widening circles. But then, there comes
a time when you start saying, "It's too much trouble to go for a swim."
Or, "Let's drive downtown. I don't feel like walking." Or, "I'd rather
stay home." You move from the big house to the smaller one. Then to
the ever-so-small and convenient condominium. As it becomes more
and more restricted, life dwindles away bit by bit, and you put yourself
into a box nature never intended for you.

Youth and beauty are always associated with kinetic behavior. Since
the quality of your life depends upon your vitality, you must accept

the fact that vitality comes from movement more than from any other single source. No matter what your age, you can reverse time's trend by moving more.

Are you worrying that exertion might be harmful? If you're a stranger to exercise, have a family history of heart ailments, are obese, smoke heavily, live on junk foods, or, in general, have a funky body, then do see a physician, preferably one who specializes in sports medicine.

Dr. Per Olof Astrand, a well-known exercise physiologist of the Swedish College of Physical Education, says, "As a general rule, moderate activity is less harmful to the healthy person than inactivity. A medical examination is more urgent for those who plan to stay inactive."

To an amazing extent, it turns out that the greater the amount of movement you exact from your body, the firmer its sense of health and well-being. Nor is this illusory. The systems of the body need work in order to stay strong and elastic. In fact, even patients with acute myocardial infarctions—for which prolonged bed rest was traditionally prescribed—are now finding themselves involved in carefully supervised physical exercise right there in the coronary-care unit, in a current experimental program. Doctors say this results in shortened hospitalization, enhanced cardiac function, and the elimination of a host of psychological and physical complications always provoked by enforced bed rest.

If you've ever broken an arm or a leg and been put in a cast, you know that immobility makes muscle tissue waste away rapidly. After the cast comes off, movement is tentative for a while, full of effort, and therefore tiring. That's a vivid analogy for what occurs very, very gradually when a body is allowed to slow down and become sedentary with age. It literally starts to wither away—although if the muscle tissue is replaced by fat the process sometimes is not visible from the outside.

What are your chances of remaining strong, vital, and full of energy when you turn seventy? Pretty good, if that's how you are at thirty. A forty-year study by Henry S. Maas and Joseph A. Kuypers, researchers from the University of California, refutes the notion that you automatically are condemned to enfeeblement as you age. They discovered, among other things, that "Old age merely continued what earlier years had launched."

□ YOUR BUILT-IN YOUTH PRESERVER

Fortunately, you have within your body one miraculous part, invisible and indivisible, which has the capability to pull you out of trouble and forestall senescence. All is not lost. You still can reactivate your built-in youth preserver. That resource is the circulatory system.

Since your heart is a muscle, exercise affects it like any other muscle that can improve and grow stronger. The improved heart muscle pumps more blood with each stroke and beats fewer times per minute. Even during exercise (or under the stress of anger or anxiety), the conditioned heart doesn't beat as rapidly as the heart that's been weakened by indolence. It returns to its "resting" rate sooner. It stands to reason that if you can strengthen your heart through saving it thousands of beats, by the time you're sixty it will show less wear and tear than if you had neglected it.

The following is a brief summary intended to encapsulate the gist of what so many medical journals report:

Regular exercise enables you to recover more quickly from stress. After a good exercise workout your bodily functions won't return at once to their poor pre-exercise level. For a while you'll continue to breathe more efficiently, your oxygen level will remain high, and you'll burn fat more steadily.

At The Golden Door we believe that the cardiovascular system is inseparable from the pulmonary system, i.e. heart and blood vessels, and lungs, and our exercises are designed to give equal emphasis to both systems, whereas most other exercise regimens ignore this relationship. Again, I'll state the case very simply: The heart and the lungs are inextricably bound in constant interplay; one cannot function effectively without the other. The oxygen your circulating blood carries is obtained through the lungs. Your heart circulates the blood through your lungs each time it goes through that familiar two-phase cycle of pump-rest, pump-rest. When your heart contracts, it forces blood through those miles of blood vessels. The contraction is followed by a rest period, and during this rest your blood fills your heart with just the right amount to be pumped out again ·in the next contraction. During exercise more blood than usual comes into the heart, which is stretched more; it then contracts more vigorously and pumps out more blood than before. This is the heart's intrinsic way of exercising its muscle.

Here is where the lungs come into play. The lungs are located within the rib cage; this chamber develops a negative pressure whenever you take in a really deep breath. The normal chest cage and lungs never have inside pressure equal to outside pressure. This negative pressure during inspiration is one of the factors helping to bring the blood back to the heart. The deeper the breath you inhale, the more negative pressure is created and the more blood comes back to your heart.

During exercise, this extraordinary coordination between your lungs and your heart becomes even more important. Because of the demands of tissue—such as those of your leg muscles when you run, or your diaphragm when you run—your requirement for oxygen and nutrients there is so much greater. More blood has to be pumped to the tissue.

The straightest route to cardiovascular/pulmonary health is to exercise for recreation and re-creation. Choose an exercise that gives you pleasure, increases your heart and respiratory rates, and causes a welcome sense of fatigue while reducing tension. With regular exercise you will recover more quickly from stress than you would if your heart weren't pumping so efficiently. Best of all, after a good workout your bodily functions won't return at once to poor pre-exercise levels.

And, if you continue to keep all systems open and functioning at full capacity, your looks will reflect the vivacity you feel.

□ WE WEREN'T BUILT TO SIT STILL

Imagine you're an apprentice historian in some distant millennium. Without any other frame of reference you are handed a microfilm of a number of ancient periodicals from a country called the United States of America, circa 1970–1980 A.D. Your assignment: Analyze the country's social structure.

Here's what you very well might write:

All riches and honors were reserved for a privileged few, called sports superstars. These individuals were treated like demigods, and great crowds gathered to cheer them in various reproductions of the Circus Maximus.

An epidemic of heart disease was sweeping the land. Medical knowledge, although crude, already had established the heart's need for exercise. Tragically, only a few were able to profit from this scientific breakthrough.

Among the citizenry a campaign had begun to claim the right to exercise in order to prolong life. But these efforts were generally spasmodic and not well organized.

The condition of the majority of the people was pathetic. At work they were cruelly confined indoors and at the end of each day's toil they were sequestered in cells from which they seldom moved.

Most fiendish of all was the practice of televising for these unfortunates scene after scene of those life-giving activities in which they were forbidden to participate.

Does that really sound so absurd?

Too many people today experience the world of sports activity only through television, newspapers, and books. To this they so easily could be adding a whole rainbow spectrum of body experience that would transform their lives.

Let me be very specific about all the rewards of exercise. You can expect payoff in the way of:

1. Psychological bonuses
2. Exorcising of tension and stress
3. Eating without stringent diets

Exercise makes you feel competent, powerful, and proud. As your self-esteem increases, you will find a parallel effect on your total lifestyle.

1. PSYCHOLOGICAL BONUSES. Taking the initiative in the matter of body movement is certain to make you feel like a winner. Exercise is the surest antidote to the poisonous miasma of mental depression, which cannot coexist with optimal physiological/psychological well-being. If you feel mental distress, and are dreading decisions, it is crucial that you avoid inertia. Move affirmatively. Whenever you feel low, get high

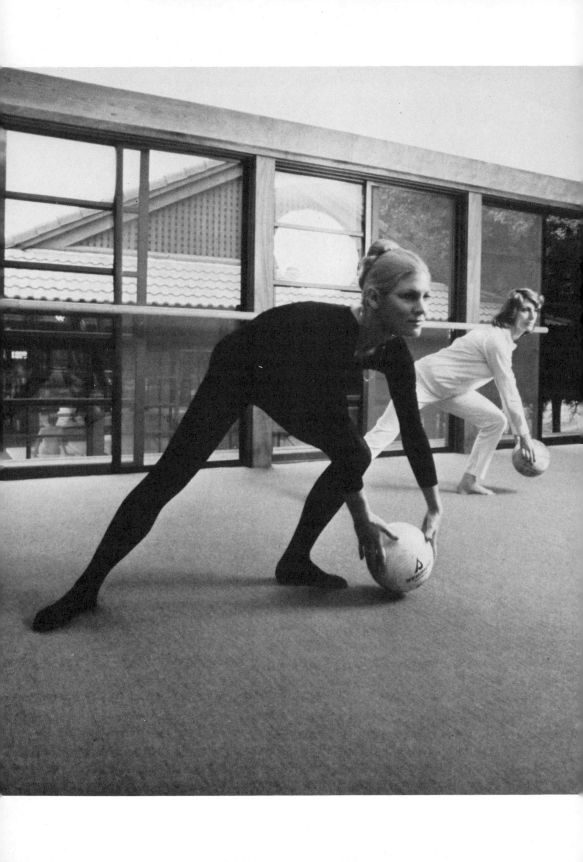

on movement. Research conducted in numerous hospitals with drug addicts and schizophrenics showed lasting improvement through marathon running—reuniting and restructuring the balance of mind and body. Many tests over the past years indicate that, after a vigorous forty-minute workout, the physiological benefits are measurable—and so is the high, which remains with you on a decreasing scale for the next six hours.

In 1970 I was a guinea pig in an early biofeedback experimentation program with Dr. Barbara Brown, renowned authority and author of *New Mind, New Body.* During those months I was hypersensitized to the relationship of mind and body, and my experiences blossomed into new insights. This was my most exciting discovery: I found that through manipulating my breathing I could also manipulate my brain waves, and I realized that breathing is a major factor in altering our states of consciousness. Therefore I believe that exercise, with its singular effect on breathing, can achieve this.

In many forms of meditation and prayer, the ritual establishes a specific, continuous breathing pattern—the Arab answering the call of his muezzin, the Jew wrapped in his prayer shawl, and the Catholic saying his beads. Sleep also has its own special breathing pattern, and ecstasy is frequently described as "breathless."

What I largely intuited then has now been confirmed in *Some Psychological Effects of Physical Conditioning,* a treatise by Dr. Thaddeus Kostrubala. This study describes an altered state of consciousness rich with intellectual associations, which are experienced as insights, and a shift in perception as the visual experience assumes a unique aesthetic importance.

Early in 1975 I had the good fortune of meeting Dr. Kostrubala, Chief of the Department of Psychiatry at San Diego's Mercy Hospital. For nineteen months he both participated in a running program and recorded his observations in his book, *The Joy of Running.* The goal of the program was to run nonstop for from forty to sixty minutes, three times a week, at 75 percent of one's maximum cardiac output. To quote from his study:

> It appears that the physical running aspects of the program act as a catalyst upon the established life patterns of the individuals . . . there

are distinct psychologic changes which occur when physiologic improvement takes place . . . decreased depression, decreased irritability and
an increasing sense of confidence and well-being . . . a reawakening of
libidinal energy . . . euphoria . . . the feeling of increased energy after
the exercise period.

This book is not prepared to teach you that kind of dedication. However, I would encourage you to read some of the new books on running,
for surely you will want to begin to run as your enthusiasm for vibrant
health increases.

2. EXORCISING TENSION AND STRESS. Several years ago we at The
Golden Door conducted a private poll of nearly a thousand supposedly
healthy upper-income people in the southwestern United States. The
large response to the poll was surprising, and so were the findings concerning tension. An overwhelming number of men and women of all
ages replied that, although they slept soundly all night, every night,
they awakened feeling physically tired. Given the busy social lives and
heavy civic and business commitments of these people, as a nonprofes-
sional analyst I found it simple to conclude that, while their minds were
continually engaged throughout the day, their bodies remained inactive.
They went to bed with minds weary from use but with bodies still
charged up and tense—no chance to reach the sweet mind-body balance
so necessary for the sort of sleep that renews. Of course I'm not the only
one who has pondered this phenomenon. A number of scientists who
have been comparing exercise with such tranquilizers as meprobamate
and alcohol say exercise wins every time.

A session of vigorous movement at the end of working hours is a
marvelous way to rid yourself of pent-up emotions. As you move, you
can give expression to all the things you couldn't say during the day.
One reason tennis has become so widely and wildly popular is that as
you hit the ball you can actually holler "Go to hell!" or whatever you've
been bursting to unburden yourself of. And even the exercise of brisk
walking gives you a chance to transform aggressions and tensions into
creative energy.

Unrelieved stress is the villain. Its relief can best be accomplished
through aggressive movement. Once you know ways to counter tension,
you needn't worry so much about high-stress situations. When the crisis
moment is past, you'll at once readjust and transmit peace hosannas to

all the parts of your body, because you will have learned how to coexist comfortably with stress. Rabindranath Tagore said it well: "Rest belongs to the work as the eyelids to the eyes."

3. EATING WITHOUT STRINGENT DIETS. Exercise allows you to enjoy your food more and also entitles you to more food to enjoy. You quite simply get to eat more than you would if you were inactive. According to metabolic law, you must balance food taken in with energy expended. So won't it be enough just to diet? Not only are most "wonder diets" masochistic, unsatisfying, and impermanent even in their superficial results, they really aren't good for you. On a strict, no-exercise diet you may be losing weight by burning off fat together with parts of your precious "lean body mass"—muscle and other nonfat tissue.

You may not even need to lose as much weight as you think. A taut body can look and feel pounds lighter. To achieve this is the main thrust of the exercise program at The Golden Door.

Abandon any fad diet you may be on and substitute common sense. Learn sensible eating, and then let exercise multiply its effects. The result: a trim figure *and* a healthy glow to show it off.

You must learn how to fine-tune your system by correlating a day's activities with the size of your meals. To help you with beauty's new math, Frank Konishi, Professor of Nutrition at Southern Illinois University, has devised a common-sense tool. His book, *Exercise Equivalents of Foods,* contains the basic information for honing down to a prettier, skinnier, more vivid You.

The Konishi book tells you how many calories are lurking within almost every kind of food imaginable. Then it lists the corresponding number of minutes of exercise—whether walking, bicycling, stepping, swimming, or jogging—you would have to put forth to burn off the calories in each food serving. Should you wish to know how many days will be required to lose a certain number of pounds, with a particular combination of calorie reduction and exercise, the book also has tables for that. Keep this little book handy in your kitchen. It can graphically and indelibly impress upon you the connection between the (food) energy input and (exercise) energy output. If you can't find the title in your bookstore, ask them to order it from Southern Illinois University Press, Carbondale, Illinois.

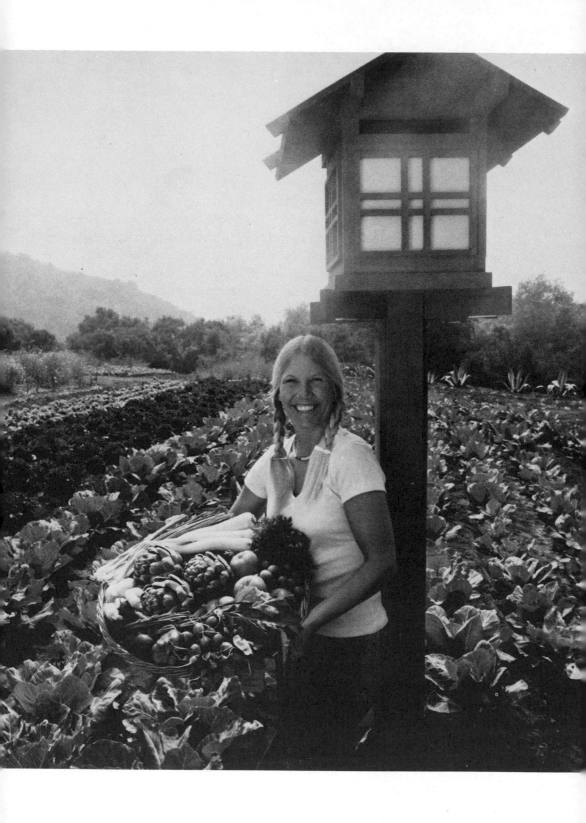

MINUTES REQUIRED AT THE EXERCISES LISTED
TO EXPEND CALORIES IN THE FOODS

FOOD	CALORIES	ACTIVITY				
		Walking Minutes	*Stepping Minutes*	*Bicycling Minutes*	*Jogging Minutes*	*Swimming Minutes*
Apple, 1 medium	87	17	12	11	9	8
Bacon, crisp, 2 slices	96	19	13	12	10	9
Banana, 1 medium	127	24	17	16	13	11
Beans, green, ½ cup cooked	15	3	2	2	2	1
Beer, 8-ounce glass	115	22	15	14	12	10
Bread and butter, 1 slice	96	18	13	12	10	9
Cake, white layer, 1⁄16 of 9" cake	250	48	33	31	25	22
Carrot, raw, 1 large	42	8	6	5	4	4
Cereal, dry, 1 cup, with milk and sugar	212	41	28	26	21	19
Cheese, American, 1-ounce slice	112	22	15	14	11	10
Cheese, cottage, 1 rounded tablespoon	30	6	4	4	3	3
Chicken, fried, ½ breast	232	45	31	28	23	21
Chicken, TV dinner	542	104	72	66	54	48
Cola beverage, 8-ounce glass	105	20	14	13	11	9
Cookie, chocolate-chip, 1 average	50	10	7	6	5	5
Cookie, vanilla-wafer, 1 average	15	3	2	2	2	1
Doughnut, 1 average	125	24	17	15	13	11
Egg, boiled or poached, 1 medium	78	15	10	10	8	7
Egg, fried or scrambled, 1 medium	108	21	14	13	11	10
French dressing, 1 tablespoon	57	11	8	7	6	5
Gelatin, with cream, 1 serving	117	23	16	14	12	10
Halibut, broiled, 1 serving	214	41	28	26	21	19

FOOD	CALORIES	ACTIVITY				
		Walking Minutes	Stepping Minutes	Bicycling Minutes	Jogging Minutes	Swimming Minutes
Ham, fresh, 2 slices cooked	254	49	34	31	25	23
Ice cream, ⅔ cup	186	36	25	23	19	17
Ice-cream soda, 1 regular	255	49	34	31	26	23
Ice milk, ⅔ cup	137	26	18	17	14	12
Malted milk, 8-ounce glass	500	96	67	61	50	45
Mayonnaise, 1 tablespoon	100	19	13	12	10	9
Milk, skim, 8-ounce glass	88	17	12	11	9	8
Milk, whole, 8-ounce glass	160	36	21	20	16	14
Milk shake, 8-ounce glass	420	81	56	51	42	38
Orange, 1 medium	73	14	10	9	7	7
Orange juice, 4-ounce glass	54	10	7	7	5	5
Pancake, 1, with 2 table- spoons syrup	204	39	27	25	20	18
Peach, 1 medium	38	7	5	5	4	3
Peach shortcake, 1 biscuit and 1 peach	266	51	35	32	27	24
Peas, green, ½ cup cooked	58	11	8	7	6	5
Pie, fruit, ⅙ of 9" pie	400	77	53	49	40	36
Pie, pecan, ⅙ of 9" pie	670	129	89	82	67	60
Pizza, cheese, ⅛ of 14" pie	185	36	25	23	19	17
Pork chop, 6 ounces raw	314	60	42	38	31	28
Potato chips, five 2" chips	54	10	7	7	5	5
Sandwiches						
Club (bacon, chicken, tomato)	590	114	78	72	59	53
Hamburger	350	67	47	43	35	31
Roast beef with gravy	430	83	57	52	43	38
Tuna salad	278	54	37	34	28	25
Sherbet, orange, ⅔ cup	120	23	16	15	12	11
Shrimp, French-fried, 3½ ounces	225	43	30	27	23	20
Spaghetti, meat sauce, 1 serving	396	76	53	48	40	35
Steak, T-bone, ½ pound raw	235	45	31	29	24	21

ENERGY COST FOR 154-POUND INDIVIDUAL, 5′9″ TALL.
If you weigh less, your caloric "costs" may be lower.
WALKING briskly at 3.5 to 4 miles per hour on the average consumes 5.2 calories
    per minute.
STEPPING 25 up and down steps per minute facing in the same direction consumes
    an average of 7.5 calories per minute.
BICYCLING consumes around 8.2 calories per minute.
JOGGING alternated with walking (5 minutes each jogging, walking, jogging, etc.)
    consumes around 10 calories per minute.
SWIMMING with average skill consumes approximately 11.2 calories per minute.

ADAPTED FROM "EXERCISE EQUIVALENTS OF FOOD," BY FRANK KONISHI, PH.D., SOUTHERN ILLINOIS UNIVERSITY PRESS (1973). USED BY PERMISSION OF FAMILY CIRCLE MAGAZINE.

□ BODY SENSE

The French use an apt phrase, *élan vital,* to express lithe, jaunty, vigorous spirits. It describes very well the inner light that emerges when people adhere to a creative exercise plan. And you don't have to go to The Golden Door to find your body sense.

The first two articles I did for *Vogue* magazine almost ten years ago were concerned mostly with rope-skipping and my fondness for it, which the editor thought very novel of me. Nobody had considered the jump rope for years, outside of fighters in training. "Jumping is a natural, undisciplined exertion," I wrote in *Vogue.* "It appeals to the child in us, and it enables us to use that child as an ally. . . . Jumping in bare feet seems to help. . . . And just *try* jumping with poor posture. . . .

"A jump rope happens to be my favorite route to huff-and-puff. I keep one in my car, my office, my briefcase, and my bedroom. It nimbles legs, upper arms, and torso, and builds up posture and stamina. Buy good solid rope from a sporting-goods store, not the lightweight variety sold in toy shops. Increase your quota of jumps and the speed with which you turn the rope with each two-minute session. . . . When to exercise? Just before meals. Before breakfast to oil away wake-up stiffness. Before lunch and dinner to soothe tensions that build up over hours of busy-ness.

Like a well-balanced mainspring, exercise both winds and unwinds, and is great before you need make an earthshaking appearance or before you embark on a dazzling evening."

Jumping rope is an easy introduction to the joys of physical activity. But as you recognize how integral movement is to the quality of a joyous life, you're going to become more and more aware of your needs for movement.

A body grows to rely on its daily movement-nourishment. Once revved up, you may note how easily you feel stifled by lack of fresh air or lack of moving around. You'll be annoyed by long periods of inactivity and will want to follow them with a brisk walk, swim, or jog. Or with the ubiquitous jump rope.

You can even turn any kind of housework into body-sculpturing exercise. Play rhythmic music while you work. Open the windows and let fresh air fill your lungs. Alternate bending-over chores with jobs that require stretching, such as washing walls.

Once you have made what I call body sense a part of your repertoire for living, you'll want to preserve its continuity, for you will find the urge to exercise (body sense) as basic an urge as appetite or thirst.

□ *VERY EASY DOES IT!*

But if you *do* fall into the trap of a long period of enforced idleness once you're an exercise regular, remember to ease yourself back into your routine, slowly.

When I was fifty I was a June bride. On our honeymoon we traveled 25,000 miles. It was an in-and-out-of-planes-cars-and-hotels month. Then, at last, we were home. To eradicate those long periods of being compressed into a tight capsule, I chose to spend my recovery day on the beach with a younger friend. We arrived mid-morning, strolled for hours along the sands, chased sand crabs and sandpipers, napped, then walked again. In the evening our husbands joined us. After picnicking we ran along the shore. At last I had stretched! At last I had breathed fully!

The next morning, I couldn't get out of bed. I had developed bursitis of the knee—which made me more than usually aware of my body, and demonstrated how easy it is to overdo.

Yes, I had behaved as gauchely as any of my most chairbound guests who, adjusting to a spa program for the first time, try too hard to catch up on activity long missed. My only excuse is that I overreacted to what I believe is an obvious "exercise instinct." Slothfulness makes me feel imprisoned, and a day without exercise seems like a day in jail. Your common sense already has persuaded you that there's no quickie approach to the joys of physical activity. Fitness depends upon fidelity to a continuing program. Exercise cannot be stored. There is a potent incentive to spur you to daily activity: the high you sustain from your new feelings of competency and attractiveness.

For primitive man, there was no question of deliberating these pros and cons of movement, nor for our forebears of one hundred or even fifty years ago. If they were to eat, they had to move. Now our environment has changed, but our bodies remain similar to those pictured in prehistoric cave drawings.

What a pity we of today have to wait till we're adults before realizing how exercise can enrich our lives. I recall a junior-high physical education instructor who blew a whistle frequently and bounced a volleyball while shouting, "Okay! Everybody out on the playground!" But at no point were we students taught the optimum exertion we need to keep in trim. Nor have my children learned it in their school.

On the other hand, children in this country are bombarded with information about their teeth. A study once proved it takes the average girl child till age eight, and a boy till twelve, to make toothbrushing automatic. As a result, whenever we walk into the bathroom we don't have to dawdle about and run through what we can remember about dental care. We just reach for the toothbrush without delay. Behind that reflex is a lot of nagging by parents, film strips in school, cards from the dentist that told you to come in and pick out a gift—and, if all else failed, there was the immediacy of a toothache and a drill-wielding dentist saying, "See? See what happens when you don't brush?"

Dental associations have done such a first-class job of public information that it's difficult to grow up in America and not know the fundamentals of home dental care. I only wish heart associations could have begun as early to broadcast their message. They might have averted what's been called the twentieth-century epidemic: coronary disease. Unfortunately it is caused by no single, easily pinpointed factor.

But topping the treacherous list of likely causes of heart degeneration is our sedentary life-style.

Ideally, we would have learned healthy movement habits in childhood. Instead, schools promote immobility. As babies and toddlers we were once lively as puppy dogs. But today the first thing we do is to send the child off to preschool, so he will learn to sit still and pay attention. The teacher plays a tune on the piano while the children walk about the room. When the music stops, each child sits on a colored dot. It is the preschool's prime achievement. Soon the child learns to grit his teeth and sit quietly throughout the entire school day—something that cannot be taught even the most well-bred chimpanzee.

☐ HOW TO PLAN YOUR PHYSICAL ACTIVITY

"You're in good shape for a man who spends his time behind the desk," I said one day to a Golden Door guest who was a member of the President's Cabinet.

"Well," he said:

> before I started coming to The Golden Door, exercise was always a catch-as-catch-can proposition. I would play golf occasionally, swim when I could, walk once in a while.
>
> But at The Door I learned the value of regularity, and particularly the value of wake-up exercise. At home I spend thirty minutes in the morning, seven days a week, right after getting out of bed, in my bedroom with the television news on. For the first ten minutes I'm on an electric bicycle, and for the next twenty I do various exercises I learned in the wake-up session that starts the day here at The Golden Door—they follow a fluid pattern from one to the next, some standing up and some on the floor.
>
> It's now such a habit that if I miss the morning exercises because of travel or tight scheduling of some sort, I don't feel right. I feel sluggish. Since I don't take the electric bicycle along when I travel, I do some extra running in my hotel room—again, while watching TV news to relieve the monotony of solo exercising.

I quote this conversation to illustrate what I always tell my guests about exercise: "Although I go to some trouble to give you guidelines for the kind of exercising I hope will be ideal for you, *I don't care how you do it, as long as you do it.*" Think of all the most efficacious exercise movements as a smorgasbord. After a little sampling you're sure to find something you want to stay with.

Best of all, try to settle on exercise that's both *isotonic* and *aerobic.*

An isotonic exercise is one that involves rhythmic, repetitive tensing and relaxing of muscles: dancing, bicycling, walking, swimming, rowing, skipping rope, working out on a mat, and so forth. The repeated squeezing of the muscles helps the blood flow and promotes cardiovascular pulmonary fitness.

An aerobic exercise is one that you can continue to perform for more than a few minutes, with oxygen being supplied to the exercising muscles all during that time. Sprinting, for example, is not aerobic because the average person can't run full blast for more than a few seconds. But all the exercises described in the chapter "Body Awakeners" (pages 96–151) are definitely aerobic.

PICK YOUR FAVORITES. You're going to be the final judge of what you and your body find likable. Together, we'll create for you a supple, bend-to-your-whim, workable schedule. The result will be a fresh pattern of movement planned especially for you and your individual life. The most wonder-working fitness trick is to make every day's physical activity into a reflex, so automatic it becomes a habit, and to smoothly fit it into its proper, most advantageous time slot.

□ *YOUR GOLDEN DOOR PLAN*

1. BEGIN THE DAY WITH A TOE-TWISTER. Do this even before you get your head together: While half-awake and vulnerable to impressions, keep your eyes closed and take a deep breath. Let it out. Take another, and let it halfway out.

Then follow the lead of Ruth West, who has written many books on food and health, and is one of the most dynamic, slender, and stylish over-sixty women I've ever known. When Ruth wakes up in her New York apartment, she exercises in bed. "That's something I learned at The Golden Door," she told me.

Exercises before I get up are marvelous because I'm too lazy to do any other kind—when I first wake up, anyway. Later, I love to walk and dance and move around a lot. But here's what I do first thing in the morning: I start with twisting my toes, turning my feet around from the ankles. Then I splay them and stretch them out. I raise and lower my legs about ten times, slowly. The next thing is what you'd just do naturally. I extend each leg alternately and stretch my arms above my head. Then I get up.

Next, Ruth performs some stretching exercises which we'll come to in a moment. "But those first little stretching exercises in bed!" she exclaims. "I couldn't start the day without them."

2. THE NAKED TRUTH. The next thing you are to do is my own special secret for reminding yourself that you're about to begin another day of living for life. It will take you just two minutes every morning.

Stepping out of bed is a propitious time for imprinting your plans and intentions for the day. Use what once was called autosuggestion. Get out of bed and stand nude, with your eyes wide open, in front of a full-length mirror. You haven't yet put on your "character armor" for the day, so you can make a very candid inventory of yourself. Stand straight and still before the mirror. Experience your Self. During two minutes of stretching, pulling, reaching, warming-up exercises, gradually mold a vision of the person you wish to be. Reproduce that image in the mirror.

Stretch each limb, one at a time, as a cat does upon waking. Rotate your head on your neck. Tuck in your chin. Elongate your spine. Stand tall. Shrug your shoulders back and forth, loosening your diaphragm and rib cage so you can feel your ribs floating high and free. Raise each knee and feel the contraction and relaxation pulse through your loins. Spread your toes and bounce on the balls of your feet.

At first, these two minutes in the morning will be a means of determining where you are. After a while you'll be using them to calculate where you want to go. And you'll become increasingly aware how productive just two well-applied minutes can be.

3. ONE STEP AT A TIME. You may have to make a few passes at settling on the program ideally suited to you. But do persist. Take things one step at a time, moving to a new goal a bit farther ahead each time you reach an older one. If you are young and very active, you may aspire to be able eventually to run a fast mile. Or you simply may want to

acquire the ability to do your very first push-up. Or to touch your fingers to the floor. Or to lose two inches off your waistline.

Take inventory at the beginning of your program, then one month later, and thereafter at three-month intervals. Of course, you can check more frequently if you perform better on a shorter leash. Whatever works and will continue to work for you is your way to go.

Two methods I have found effective are:

a. Tricks of a Ten-Percenter—for the person who already is fairly active

b. An Hour a Day Keeps the Doctor Away

a. *Tricks of a Ten-Percenter.*   If you're in your twenties or thirties and have one specific bulge you wish to erase, being a ten-percenter will probably suffice. Odds are high that you run and jump and dance and play often enough to keep your circulatory system perking. With just a bits-and-pieces exercise program, you soon will stand taller, be trimmer, and whip about with better muscle tone.

Ask yourself how you can slyly insert 10 percent more movement into all the normal activities of your day, adding just a little here and there. Park your car blocks away from your appointment and walk. Step off the elevator a few floors below the one you want and walk up the stairs.

The ten-percent route is a particularly good way to reach some of the parts of your body that tend to get lost and never receive any workouts: If tension localizes in your neck during the day, for example, you can use the wait at a stoplight to roll your head in a circle or do some loosening exercise you find relaxing.

On shorter errands, use a bicycle instead of a car. Park at the far end of the shopping center's lot. Carry your own groceries to your bike or car, or all the way home if you don't live too far away—a task you can lighten by shopping every other day for crisp dewy-fresh foods instead of packing home a huge load once a week (see "Glorious Eating," page 170).

People in offices ought to replace the coffee break with a movement break. It's a change of pace your body silently craves, more than it wants a prune Danish, a cigarette, or coffee. So walk quickly around the block. Or jump rope through the building corridors (any glances that come your way will be ones of envy). Once you have begun to enjoy yourself, every activity at home or work will trigger some extra exercise idea. And you'll be in shape before you know it.

b. *An Hour a Day Keeps the Doctor Away.* It's my fervent belief that the basic requirement for your well-being and good looks is a daily hour of exercise. However, you can get by on forty minutes a day (but no less) at least three times a week. Try for five times, Monday through Friday, to allow some leeway for the occasional rainstorm or breakfast meeting—and if you can steal time from the weekend, so much the better.

Golden Door graduates return to their homes with an exercise plan that comes in two styles: one for the person who likes to complete most of a day's work before noon (I also recommend this as a solution for the hate-to-get-up type), and the other for the person who needs extra help in untwisting the knots at the end of the day. We all require some exercises for both getting up and getting down.

The Morning Pattern—Winding Up: Forty minutes of springy exercise and hard breathing, including a few minutes for warm-up and cool-down, as part of your breakfast time can point you toward a nice clear high. A brisk walk-jog is a joyous beginning. Or practice some of the exercises shown later in this book. Afterward, you'll absolutely float through the day. Then you'll require a refresher of twenty more minutes of exercise (at twilight).

The Evening Pattern—Winding Down: The pattern for the evening person is the mirror opposite of the morning. If your day is taut with high-tension situations, you may have no trouble getting up for it but you will have trouble settling down later. The best way to approach such a day is to start before breakfast with twenty minutes of vigorous exercise. The important forty-minute stint will come at twilight, before dinner. This is a life-saver for people whose days call up a lot of fight-or-flight reflexes which release all the adrenaline without giving it any place to go. Tension with no place to go is diverted inward, where it becomes hostile to the mind/body (thus the tension headache, the back pain, the indigestion, and the ulcers).

I'm convinced that for most adult Americans the standard twilight exercise, the evening's drink or drinks, is a response to their recognition that they must do something to untense. You know as well as I the many reasons why alcohol is essentially bad for people. But let me provide you with one more (which I hope will lead you to a momentous, life-extending decision to first limit your alcoholic intake to wine—and eventually to give it up altogether). The problem with alcohol is that it relaxes you entirely too well, and is a depressant. You have two drinks, deactivate yourself, and manage to retain barely enough spark to sink into a comfortable armchair with a magazine or in front of the television.

Here is the result: To the degree and with the rapidity that your blood sugar zooms, within an hour or so (depending on your movement pattern and evening meal) there will be an equivalent *drop*.

What do you do, then, for a pickup at the end of your day's work? Before you leave your place of business, or a half-hour before dinner, nibble on a healthful blood-sugar builder: a cup of hot broth and just a small piece of cheese eaten slowly; or a few raisins and sunflower seeds and a small apple. Within thirty or forty minutes, when your body has had time to react to these energy-boosters, you will feel a surge of energy. Advise yourself this is going to happen and be ready to notice that zinger of vitality when it strikes.

MIX AND MATCH. Mix and match elements from the basic approaches. You may wish to add two minutes of rope-jumping to your showering and makeup time in the morning; *and* walk to the market every day; *and* reserve half an hour before dinner to put a twilight twinkle into your eye. Fine, so long as you remember to include at least one real segment of sustained exertion somewhere in your daily plan.

Draw up a list of
1. Different kinds of exercises and sports
2. Exercise classes available where you live
3. Physical chores you perform around your home

Rate them by dividing them into three categories: the ones you like very, very much; those you can tolerate; and what you cannot stand. Select accordingly. It's your plan, intended to last you a lifetime, so let it reflect your personality and style. Improvise. Observe your own reactions (may they be joyous).

In time, like a Washington, D.C., journalist I know, you may make up your own rules. She gave a dinner in my honor on one of my regular autumn trips to the East, and I couldn't refrain from remarking how slim and marvelous she looked. She had undergone a becoming weight change since we first met. Her husband raised his glass to both of us. "To Deborah," he said. "You've changed my life. Among other things, I know that it's morning when my wife is wearing her blue jogging suit, and that it's bedtime when she's in her red leotard. The only difference between our house and Stillman's Gym is that our place smells better."

Red leotard at bedtime? I must have looked puzzled. "I'm on the evening pattern," my reporter friend explained, "but with one twist— I do half an hour of spot exercises just before going to bed." (Many of them are similar to the Body Awakeners shown on pages 104–140.)

"I know you say they should be done to music but since we have no record player upstairs in our bedroom I watch television to amuse myself. It doesn't get me too pepped up to go to bed, as it does some people. I'll sit down for ten minutes or so afterward, then go straight to bed, and I'm ready for sleep."

The early-morning part of her day's activity consists of a mile-and-a-quarter jog before breakfast. It takes her about twelve minutes. (At the time of her first visit to The Golden Door three years before she had never jogged; as of last year, her husband joins her and runs three miles a day.)

> I walk a great many places I never would have before. I hop a cab only when it's too far to go and I don't have time to walk it. And after my last trip to The Golden Door I skied better and longer than I ever dreamed possible. I just have a lot more stamina, a lot more fun now because of the constant exercise—and because I'm thinner.

Another guest tells me that what she does at the office and elsewhere is to walk up and down stairs wherever she can find them. In an elevator culture, that occasionally arouses some peculiar looks. The last time she was in Chicago, staying on the eighth floor of a hotel, she found the stairs after much searching and started walking up and down them. The hotel maintenance people who used the stairs began to recognize her. One day, as she passed the third floor, one of the men opened the door for her, thinking she was a run-of-the-mill guest going from one floor to another. Then he took a second look and said, "Oh, that's right, you're *that* one!"

I would guess that anticipation makes exercising twice the work: once when you think about it and again when you do it. Don't think about it. Do it.

□ *INSPIRE THE CHILD WITHIN*

FIND FELICITOUS, IMAGINATIVE SURROUNDINGS. You choose to dine in pretty restaurants rather than eating in dull and dreary surroundings. Why not similarly stage-design your physical activity?

Do you have a nearby park with greenery and knolls and winding paths and a soft springy turf? Use it. Explore all of it. Why jog around only the edge, next to the exhaust fumes? To have fresh air, sunshine, and living grass and trees around us is always a treat for the senses under any circumstances.

Do you have a garden of your own? Use it as a background for exercising. You can use the natural perfume of all outdoors to reactivate your breathing apparatus. If you're a city dweller and you're generally confined indoors, the plant shop on your block can help you bring the world of nature into your apartment.

When exercising indoors choose your largest room, preferably one with large windows, and open them all the way. If furniture is cramping you, move it aside. You want space in which to breathe deeply and to kick out all the kinks.

USE MUSIC TO ORCHESTRATE YOUR EXERCISES. Music creates good feeling and keeps movement flowing naturally. At first, just put on your favorite music as background. Later you can start moving in tempo with the beat. The advantage, beyond the sheer euphony of it all, is that music can cue you to what exercise movement comes next.

REWARD YOURSELF. Chances are you don't receive nearly as much physical attention as you did when you were six years old—yet the child within you still adores it. You can harness that feeling to motivate yourself, in the same way that The Golden Door helps guests persevere in some very tough routines. We supply various "strokes" as lavish reward for hard work. Arranged around Japanese gardens and courtyards are salons replete with massages and facials and herbal wraps.

One distinguished psychoanalyst told me he was outraged by these "decadent frills"—that is, until the end of his first day when, as he sank with relief onto the massage table, he realized how richly he deserved to be stroked and catered to like a king. He had earned it. Your rewards to yourself needn't be elaborate. If you can afford to install a sauna, a steam cabinet, or a Japanese hot tub, don't hesitate. Any of these will beautifully soothe your hardworking body. But just an occasional facial or beauty treatment can make you feel as if you've been decorated with honors.

Not all the payoffs need be physically therapeutic. A ticket to a concert, an afternoon off for window-shopping, or a long-postponed tea with some friends are other ways of telling your psyche, "Congratulations!"

SHARE WORKOUTS WITH FRIENDS, OLD AND NEW.   Doing anything with a friend intensifies the experience, so enroll together in a class in dance-exercise, or form one. Your initial aches and eventual triumphs should be shared with others who are like-minded. A special sort of fellowship often develops among such classmates, and you may find your life expanding with new friends as you wonder how you ever managed without them. You can swap exercise ideas, lighten occasional moments of gloom—and applaud each other's progress.

☐ *IMAGERY AND EXERCISES*

Your body finds joy in a spectrum of movement. That's why our Body Awakeners have been designed to move and stretch every inch of you and to awaken your appetite for sampling the world of exercise activity.

Let imagination lift you: Focus on the sensations within your body whenever you exercise. You are going to appreciate them more and more. Since the act of seeing distracts your attention from your body, from time to time close your eyes as you move. Occasionally you may wish to go through some movements in slow motion, concentrating on the muscles that control the movement, and relaxing others.

Try these four visualizations:

1. FEEL THE FORCE OF GRAVITY.   The most efficient and graceful movement occurs when your muscles and bones are perfectly aligned with

gravity as they go about their work. Another word for this is *balance.* Feel for balance as you move. Flex forward and back and sideways as you exercise, until you reach that central point of balance where all your forces are aligned with gravity and none is being dissipated in the strain of misalignment.

2. MOVE FROM YOUR CENTER.   The big muscle masses that should take care of your heavy work are located close to the vertical axis of the body, the spine. When you stand sideways to the mirror, ideally you want your ears, the tips of your shoulders, your hipbones, and your anklebones to line up. You win a bonus in balance when they do, as well as an easy elegant posture that is admired for itself alone.

Imagine that every movement of your arms and legs is initiated by the spine. You'll discover that you now are in *perfect* balance, using muscles close to your core.

3. MOVE LENGTHWISE.   All muscles have to contract to do their work, but some tend to remain contracted even when not working. These produce extra tension which the working muscles have to fight against, reducing the body's efficiency.

Many people don't even know that the muscles of the neck near the shoulders are usually contracted and tense. As you run or work out, imagine a string is attached to the top of your head, pulling upward and gently stretching your spine, elongating your body. Drop your shoulders. Focus on your spine and loosen all the muscle groups that are binding it, shortening it, and stiffening it. Soon you'll feel a stretching, lengthening effect that is also a new relaxation.

4. MOVE LIGHTLY.   Here's another example of the interaction of mind and body. Point your elbows down and hold them firmly in position as a friend puts her hands under them and tries to lift you off the ground. You can make yourself seem lighter to her by visualizing yourself as weightless, as part of a current of energy pouring up and through you toward the sky. But if you picture yourself as inert, she'll have a great deal more trouble lifting you.

Obviously, you always can make your movement seem light and buoyant by picturing yourself that way. This is just another facet, just another quality of excellence, of vitality, that exercise can add to your life.

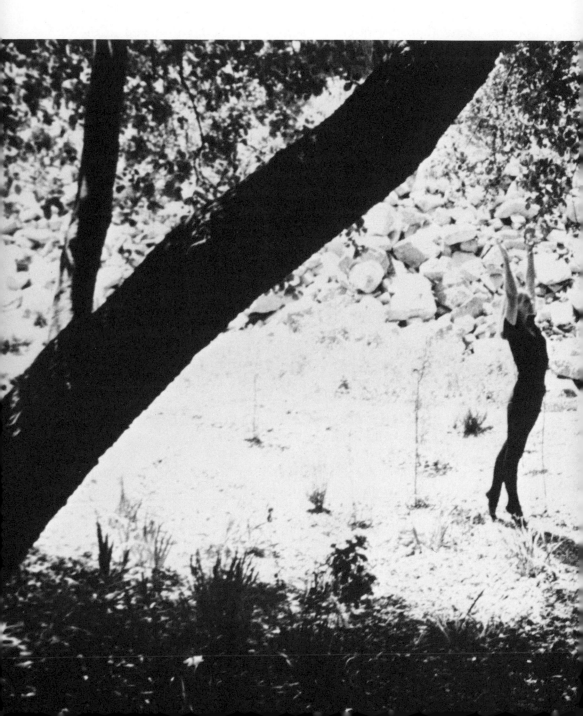

CHAPTER III

BODY AWARENESS: ANOTHER SOURCE OF BEAUTY

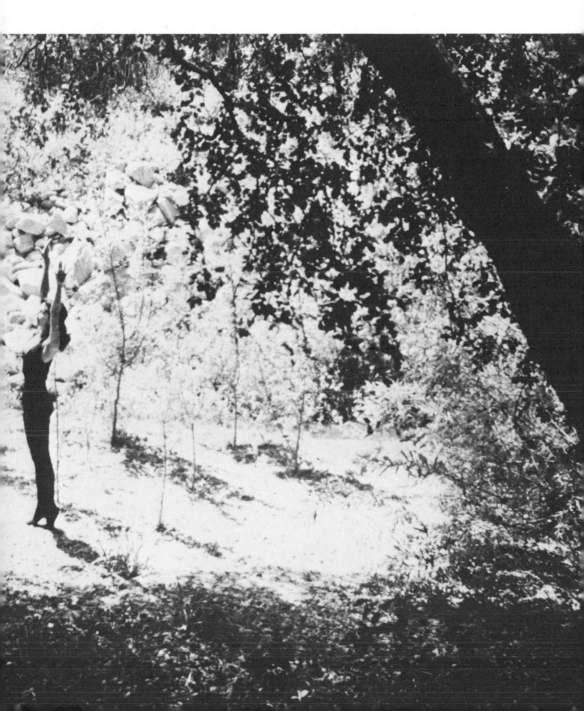

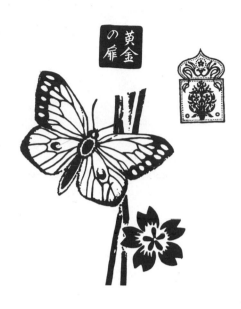

THERE IS A SAYING THAT ALL BRIDES ARE BEAUTIFUL, AND IT'S TRUE, because for a little while, the young woman being married has everyone's permission to focus all her attention on herself. I have never seen a bride approach an altar with bad posture. It is this ability to be aware of herself that separates an attractive woman from a plain one.

You can keep your own excitement alive even though you are not a bride. Listen to your senses. That is the first step in this exciting journey that you and I have set out upon. You have a whole new world to explore, full of unknown resources and inspirations. It starts at your skin and proceeds inward.

Your body wants to feel healthy. Your muscles are eager to move. If you will open up your senses to learn what your body is trying to tell you, you will find it your most reliable guide. The fact is, true health and beauty come from no external source; they come from within yourself. When you look into the new world under your skin, you will find that exploring it will be the greatest adventure you have ever known.

Your only guide should be what makes you feel good. You have already made a big move in the direction of feeling fine by choosing the first essential of well-being—regular physical activity. But don't rely on sheer willpower alone to make your exercise last a lifetime. There are two marvelous additional essentials available to you—relaxation and joy.

Instead of drifting thoughtlessly through your physical activities, become newly aware of your body as you let your movements be guided and personalized by your senses. Make contact with the flow of feelings that

1. ensures that your daily activities are adapted to the needs of *your* life and *your* body;

2. helps you to banish tension and feel the full benefits of exercise;

3. opens a whole new realm of delightful sensations that expand, enrich, and sustain your health and beauty program.

Soon you will notice that you have plenty of company, because, as you experience your senses and your body awakens, as your skin begins to glow and your eyes to sparkle, others around you will share the same excitement. In some mysterious way, people who delight in themselves delight others as well.

☐ EXPERIENCING YOUR BODY

In recent years there has been an explosion of information about food, exercise, and health in general. How do you judge what is valid? How can you choose what is healthy for you?

Amid all the conflicting advice, there is one way, and one alone, for you to know what is good for you. Listen to your body. Pay attention to what your senses are telling you. Awareness of breathing, muscle tension, skin sensations, heartbeat—these and other interior processes, as well as good elimination, sound sleep, and hearty appetite, are your key checkpoints.

It is not difficult. I'm not asking you to achieve the kind of total control over the body that a yogi has. What I want you to do is to get to know yourself and to bring balance into your sensory world by listening to what your body is telling you. For years, your messages have come from "out there"; now you are going to spend some time listening to "in here."

Have you been a puritan up to now? Have you been one of those people who are afraid that too much sensuality will distract them from higher intellectual or spiritual pursuits, who insist that there are more important things in life than pampering the body? Believe me, a healthy body, over whose workings you have control, will never hinder you from striving for these higher goals. Indeed, a sound body is the greatest aid to freeing your mind. It puts *you* in control and lets you make the choices.

Making contact with a long-dormant body presents some people with forms of excitement they hadn't counted on. Blair Sabol, one of the busiest writers in America, who often writes on fashion and beauty, used to pay some attention to her body, mostly by doing stretches and bends whenever she thought of it. After her first visit to The Golden Door, she found herself paying more attention to aerobics and to the feedback her body gives her, so she takes a morning walk on the beach when she can—"but there are times when that's hard for me, especially if I stay out past twelve o'clock the night before."

"What I *do* manage to do," she said, "every single day in Los Angeles, is to take an exercise class." She went on:

> . . . an hour and a half of huffy-puffy work. I have the kind of body that has to move a lot before I feel anything, so this class is like a bunch of Body Awakeners all in a row.
>
> It's a damned nuisance, to be frank. I have to take it early in the morning or late in the evening so I can construct a day around it. But it's my therapy. A lot of my friends are going to shrinks, and I'm putting the time and money toward getting to know my body. Maybe I'm getting as much as they are; we'll see.

She barely paused for breath before the rush of words continued.

> I did find one thing about The Door that was disconcerting. You know, by the middle of the week I found myself doing all the movement, eating the food with gusto, feeling absolutely terrific about myself. My body got revved up—and then, a week or two after I left The Door, something happened—a big mental drop.
>
> I had just experienced myself being in the best shape I'd ever been in, as if every muscle was cleaned and toned and sparkling, and for once I knew what it must feel like to be an athlete.

Blair decided that the problem lay in going home to the old stimuli that made old habits want to come back. She sees her walk and the exercise class as ways to hold on to The Golden Door experience.

Awareness of the way her body feels, however, comes to Blair's rescue even when it isn't entirely comfortable.

> I figured out that I can do a lot of little things as triggers for my Door experience every day out here in the real world. That's why I try to do something every day that reminds me of The Door. The walk, the exercise class, tricks with food. If I miss two days in a row of that exercise class, I start feeling the slippage. . . . I am plagued with the fear that I'm addicted to The Door.

□ *YOUR MESSENGERS: THE SENSES*

All your knowledge about the world and about your body comes to you, of course, through your sensory systems, so let's examine them briefly. As you read and experience these sensations, contemplate the miracles that lie within your body; it is as much an energy center as is the universe, and it is yours to direct.

We all have not just the traditional five senses of sight, hearing, taste, smell, and touch. We actually have seven. The extra two are kinesthesia (the sense of position and movement in the body) and balance (provided by the inner ear).

I call kinesthesia and balance, along with touch from among the traditional five senses, the "body" senses, since they provide you with information about what is going on *inside* your body. Just because they aren't "head" senses like the first four—that is, they aren't used primarily to provide information about what is happening out in the world—you must not forget to cultivate them.

Take a look at the two extra senses, kinesthesia and balance.

KINESTHESIA. This real sixth sense is at least as complex and mysterious as ESP, the supposed "sixth sense" that some researchers are convinced we can develop. For a simple demonstration of kinesthesia, close your eyes and touch your nose with a fingertip. Now think: How do you know that your finger is moving toward your nose?

You have millions of nerve endings with specialized sense organs built into all the muscle tissue of your body. As each muscle tenses and relaxes, complex messages are transmitted to your brain, which "charts" the progress of the movement being made.

There are not only nerve hookups to the voluntary skeletal muscles; we also receive information from the heart, from the muscles that push our food through the intestines, and from other muscles which do all the other routine work of the body. The result is that we have the potential for knowing what is happening anywhere within our bodies at any given moment. The same nervous system tells us how much strain each muscle is undergoing.

The formal word for the nerve endings that give you such important bodily information is *interoceptors.*

BALANCE. Besides these interoceptors, our bodies have a remarkable organ that lets us know how we are placed and in what direction we are going relative to the ground. It is, of course, the inner ear that provides us with a sense of balance and orientation.

SENSE-STRETCHING. Because all seven senses are at your command, your body is a marvelously flexible device. Remember, your body was designed to be used in a broad array of ways. You need not restrict yourself to a narrow range of movement and sensation.

If you are feeling stale, your problem is not one of sloth. I do not believe that you are lazy, and that you indolently lie around the house all day doing nothing. But you might be leading a "steady-state" life; that is, you might be moving through the same repetitive daily activities, almost as though you had been programmed, so that the muscles and the senses you haven't been using are sluggish.

We have learned at The Golden Door to alternate between vigorous exercise and voluptuous relaxation, not just to give hardworking bodies a rest but also to open up the whole thrilling range of awareness that is available to everyone. Just as some movements are designed to awaken your muscles, so relaxation allows your senses to move into new, undiscovered freedom.

Discover for yourself your own repertoire of sense-stretchers. A good way to start is to give yourself a chance to exercise your awareness as consciously as you exercise your muscles. If you can take a whole day off, fine. If not, make a quiet place within your day, an hour or two if you can. But remember, you are setting aside this time for you to do things for *yourself,* not for others. Ignore any charges of vanity or selfish-

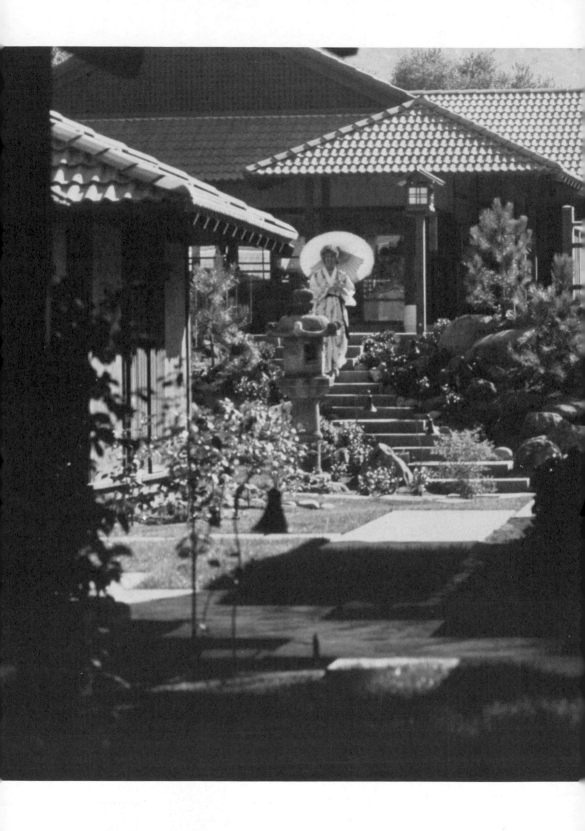

ness as you find ways and make the time to do these awareness exercises.

SIGHT.   Strive for a broad range of visual input, long-range and close-up, quick-scanning and point-watching. Caress a variety of visual textures with your eyes. Trace crisp outlines and bright colors in strong sunshine; in duskiness, soften your focus and pay attention to the masses and backgrounds of your visual field. At night, turn out some of the lights in your living room to create some contrast between areas of darkness and pools of brightness.

Here are four specific exercises to relax and freshen the eyes. Repeat each one as often as you can without discomfort.

1. *Eye Painting.*   Stand relaxed with your arms hanging loosely. Begin swinging your body from side to side. When you feel secure, close your eyes for a few seconds, then open them partly so that the world is just a blur passing by. Finally open your eyes completely, without focusing. Swing your eyes right to left, then left to right. Imagine your sweep of vision as a paintbrush making horizontal strokes. Just enjoy the shapes and color impressions flashing by, without trying to give them meaning or outline.

2. *Range-Switching.*   If you are reading or doing other close work, periodically look up and out at some distant object, giving your eyes a break by changing the focal length of the lens. Switch back and forth from close up to far away.

3. *Blinking.*   It breaks the strain of looking steadily. Simply blink in a slow, regular rhythm, concentrating on the muscles around the eyes, relaxing them, getting rid of squinting and other tensions. Vary the speed next, moving to a rapid flutter.

4. *Eyeball Rolling.*   Rotate your eyes in their sockets, not too hard. Go clockwise, then counterclockwise, trying to catch the shadows that are made at the peripheries by your eyelids.

HEARING.   Aim for the same kind of contrast you gave your eyes. Focus on the smaller sounds that are normally drowned in the blast of traffic and household noise: crickets, the closing of a window, or the soft susurrus of a breeze in the trees.

TASTE.   We need never worry about the tongue muscle being under-exercised. Seldom is it idle. It works hard to help us speak and is even more industrious at mealtime. The tongue performs a muscular marathon, pushing food back beyond the teeth, mixing food with saliva, then helping push the food back for swallowing (a function which it performs even when we humans are in the fetal state). See also "Glorious Eating" (page 170) and the recipes at the back of the book.

SMELL. Seek out the less strident odors. Perfume your sheets so that when you go to bed you can imagine yourself submerged in deep, soft fragrance. Place scents in handbags, dress linings, anywhere that will give pleasure to you and those around you. Surround yourself with flowers, a few growing plants, and a touch of incense now and then. Be aware of the dry scent of rocks baking under the sun, of newly mowed lawns, of baking bread, of fresh new breezes—there are hundreds of lovely smells we take for granted.

TOUCH. You probably know that the skin is a single, complex organ —the largest of all our organs. Forming the physical boundary of our selves, it contains one of the most basic sensory systems, the sense of touch. Touch has been called the "mother of senses" because it develops in the embryo earlier than any other sense.

Notice that when you really want to verify the existence of something, you want to touch it. Lovers are always touching each other. Touching, in short, is one of the basic ways to communicate emotion, and we all need our quota of caresses, given and received.

On a less emotional level, you can greatly increase your awareness of the sheer information that comes to you through your skin. A few of the areas are:

Texture. Think how much poorer your life would be if you could never distinguish the difference in texture between moss, grasses, a handful of rich loam, or autumn leaves. Try sleeping nude and be conscious of the sleek sheets and their cool folds against your body.

Pressure. Have you ever played the game in which someone writes on your back with a finger while you try to decipher the message? The skin is amazingly sensitive to variations in pressure. When you step from your bath, play afterbath pat-a-cake, giving yourself gentle pats all over at a moderately brisk tempo, just before toweling off. Pat with one finger, with a flat hand, with cupped hands, and use varying degrees of force. After a little such conditioning, you'll react to even the subtlest distinctions in pressure.

Temperature and Humidity. The touch of the air upon the skin when you step outdoors tells you whether the atmosphere is balmy or frigid, muggy or arid. The next time you reach into the oven, notice that just for an instant you can detect the boundary between the hot air inside and the cold air outside. Vary the temperature of your shower: from warm to hot, to very hot, to cool, to icy cold.

□ **YOUR POSTURE:
A GAUGE OF KINESTHESIA
AND BALANCE**

To remind yourself of the precision with which you can enjoy kinesthesia and balance, go back to the chapter on movement and run through the four visualizations of feeling the force of gravity, moving from your center, moving lengthwise, and moving lightly. As you practice each one, observe how you hold yourself during the exercise and also later while sitting, standing, resting, and performing everyday routines. It's your body alignment that you're regarding now with a critical eye.

The next time you watch your body move, have in mind these little secrets of proper alignment:

1. As you stand tall, squeeze your buttock muscles tautly.

2. While walking, pretend you're carrying a jug of water on each shoulder and you will have to go back to the well if the water spills.

3. Pretend you're a night-running locomotive. There's a powerful light shining from the center of your chest, boring through the blackness. Your job is to keep the beam aimed straight at the track ahead.

Your posture continually sends messages in two directions. Inwardly, it reports the ways your body responds to gravity, to the muscular demands of any task you set yourself, and to your state of mind. All of this influences your vitality. Distorted posture means your muscles can't work efficiently, and your energy is being sapped as muscle groups struggle against one another instead of cooperating.

Outwardly, posture is your body's statement about how vital and attractive and strong you feel. If you permit your stomach muscles to go too slack, your spine will curve and a "pot" will protrude in front.

Shoulders also will slope forward to compensate, the chin will drop, and wrinkles and double chins will form. Your carriage always is sending a distinct message about you to the world outside.

I grew up with dreadful posture—a tendency to hunch my head forward. I'm convinced it was because of an attitude toward life I developed when I was very young. Today I have improved my posture sufficiently not to mind talking about it.

As the first child I took on a good deal of responsibility very early in life. My mother refused to take care of household finances; my father would give me a check and, from the time I was thirteen, I budgeted for us all. Then came marriage at seventeen and the responsibility of running Rancho La Puerta and handling dozens of staff people, some of them two or three times my age. It all added up to my feeling that the world was sitting on my back. I became more and more hunched.

Someone more timid than I might have pushed her nose ahead of her like a rabbit; another, more defensive, might have pulled her head in like a turtle. It's hard to be outgoing and expansive if you have the stance of either a rabbit or a turtle.

The first step in changing ourselves is often a matter of changing our posture. If you can stand tall and loose, head up and feet well planted, you feel—and look—like a person centered between the earth and the skies. Good posture is particularly important as one grows older because bad posture inhibits breathing. You need the full capacity of your lungs to supply oxygen to your brain. So sit and stand *tall*. This will directly affect your behavior and the response of everyone you meet.

Through kinesthesia and balance there are several ways to build a simple, erect, and efficient stance. Try these:

1. THE MARIONETTE. I like the image of a strong, invisible silken cord pulling me up from the solar plexus, through to the center of my head, as if I were a puppet on a string. To imagine the tug of the cord, the stretch, the upward trend, will make me elongate my body line every time I think of it.

2. YOUR DIAPHRAGM AS A CONCERTINA. I always remember to stand tall when I think of my diaphragm as a concertina I can expand and stretch wa-a-ay out, just as an accordionist does when he performs.

3. BONESTACKING. Your bones are designed to carry the weight of your body; your muscles, to move it. But when the skeleton's alignment

is all out of kilter, the muscles have to do support duty as well and you're going to feel tired in a hurry.

In your mind, try to picture each bone. Tell yourself to feel how each portion of the bone structure rests solidly on the one below. Be aware of gravity passing vertically through your whole body frame.

4. ELIMINATING VISUAL INPUT. Close your eyes and stand straight, arms held out to the sides at right angles. Lift one knee above your waist and try to hold it there for ten seconds. Equalize the muscle tensions all over your body. Don't let them localize—you'll topple.

Take other positions while you stand with your eyes closed and rely completely on your kinesthetic sense.

5. THE BODY PLEDGE OF ALLEGIANCE. My reflection in a looking-glass or a shop window makes me think of my morning exercise time (and that full-length mirror) and draw myself up. That's why in looking at photographs of myself today and thirty years ago I see such a marked difference in my posture. I now have a posture that proclaims my happiness. People who haven't seen me for many years always say, "You've lost weight!" (I haven't.) Or they exclaim, "You look so much younger!" (I am not.)

□ SENSORY UNDERLOAD

You must provide yourself with contrast and change in order to function with all systems at go. But, exactly as too little activity can cause the senses to atrophy, so can too much. You'll simply blank out if you're bombarded too steadily with an overload of stimuli.

For refreshment you need occasional periods of sensory *under*load. For one day, or even two or three, give your taste buds a rest with the Virtue-Making Diet (page 205). From time to time, sit for half an hour in silence. Turn out the lights at twilight and rest your eyes in the dusty-lilac dusk. Turn off.

Dr. John Lilly, who became celebrated for his research with dolphins, has carried the concept of sensory deprivation to its logical extreme in his experimental work. Inside his "Lilly tank"—a container of salty body-temperature water—a human research subject floats with eyes and ears covered, and nothing at all to touch. Subjects report that, as senses go into eclipse, their inner imagery and other forms of consciousness shoot off on new and sometimes unexpected tangents.

□ HOW INNER COMMUNICATIONS ARE SHORT-CIRCUITED

Although the three "body" senses (touch, balance, and kinesthesia) also enable us to know our physical selves in almost infinite detail, most of the information flowing through our skin and interoceptors never gets through to consciousness. Somewhere along the line it is shut out.

For example, how often are you aware of your digestion? Most of us know nothing about what is happening in our intestines unless a gross disorder occurs and a red-flagged message finally gets through.

There are two barriers to perfect communication via the body senses. Luckily, both can be overcome. The first is merely lack of education. Many of us are sensory illiterates who never were taught to be aware of our skin, our motions, and our balance. The remedy lies in simple exercises such as those in this chapter. The second barrier is tension. Many of us have learned to shut off the sometimes painful flow of information from the body. We do this by muscle-clenching. This powerful inhibitor of our body senses is the state doctors call stress and most of us call tension.

□ THE DIS-EASE OF TENSION

After years of considering my problems and those of my guests, together we have learned that treating the symptoms of stress is nowhere near as effective as finding ways to develop ease and adroitness in the ways you handle stress. If you're a high achiever with an exciting life, you live with stress. There has to be some of it in every life, but you definitely can learn how to convert tension to creative action.

Tension is basically a physiological reaction to emotion. Whenever a person entertains fear or rage, the body prepares itself for action. Blood pressure rises, pulse and heartbeat quicken, body temperature goes up, digestion slows down, adrenaline pours into the bloodstream. More sugar is then manufactured to feed energy to the muscles. The muscles themselves tighten—and there you have tension buildup.

□ *IDENTIFYING TENSION*

Virtually everyone has his or her own body signature—a personal pattern of tension that produces an individual posture and gait.

Try this experiment: Lie down on the floor, on your back, and relax. If you are truly relaxed, almost all of your spine will touch the floor except for a few vertebrae in the small of your back. If you have tension in the lower back, a common place for it, your spine will arch away from the floor.

Now, while you are still relaxed and on your back, your arms lying slack with the palms down, raise the fingers of your left hand as high as you can. Just bend your wrist back, nothing else. Focus your attention on the upper forearm and the muscle there that you clenched to bend your wrist. Feel the muscle with your mind; that is the sensation of tension. Get to know it, so you can recognize it elsewhere in your body.

Some other very common centers of tension are:

1. Forehead and scalp: Tense muscles here are major contributors to headaches and eye aches.

2. Jaw: Tooth-grinding and clenching of the jaw can cause pain.

3. Nape of neck: Another contributor to headaches, fatigue, and general feelings of rigidity.

4. Shoulders: A great fatigue-producer; tension here easily spreads to the neck and produces a headache.

5. Stomach and abdomen: Tension here is often associated with ulcers (although it does not cause them directly).

6. Buttocks and anus: Colon disorders are a possible result of chronic tension here.

No matter where the tension is, you will know it by its pain—a headache, a dull muscle ache that is quite different from the twinge you might feel in a muscle you just used for the first time in months—and by the most reliable indicator, fatigue. You know the fatigue I mean—not the pleasant tiredness of an exercised body, but the draggy feeling you wake up with after what should have been a good night's sleep.

□ *EXERCISES TO DISSOLVE TENSION*

Return to your position on the floor, on your back. Strain your left wrist backward just as you did before. Let your hand fall back to the floor, of its own weight. Now feel the forearm, in your mind. Don't make an *effort* to relax. Real relaxation is neither trying nor doing; rather, it's doing nothing. The forearm muscle feels very different now, doesn't it? Can you sense the increased flow of blood and easy energy? That's the sensation of relaxation.

You can apply the same principle to every muscle group in your body. For *gradual relaxation,* you add one extra series of steps: Instead of progressing from full tension to full relaxation in just one jump, do it in stages. Start with that same left arm. Tense it slightly, then a little more and a little more, until after ten seconds the arm has reached maximum rigidity. Now relax in the same small stages, back down to your original limp state. And then concentrate on relaxing your arm even further. Keep on letting go.

If you progressively relax all your muscles in this way, you'll soon be adept at recognizing residual tension and releasing it. Monitor the different muscle groups. Grow familiar with the areas most vulnerable to stress. At various times throughout the day, check to be sure you're not tightening up.

There's another way to vary tension systematically. If you discover a section of your body tensed, try *shaking* it loose. First the hands and arms, then shoulders and head, feet and legs; finally shimmy the entire body. Now relax and feel that tingle.

Muscular contraction is just one of the hints your body gives you about tension buildup. Another is shallow, inhibited breathing. The flow of feeling parallels the flow of breath. If you doubt that, notice how you breathe the next time you're confronted by danger or a need for quick action: Your breath crowds into the top half of your chest as part of the fight-or-flight mechanism.

It's impossible to experience your body totally when you're breathing in shallow little gasps. But when you breathe fully and deeply, the body acknowledges a signal that all is safe. Tension drains off, and sensations and feelings flow freely.

That's why almost every mental and physical discipline begins with exercises in *breath control.* The ancient Hindus revered breath as so precious that they spoke of the measure of human life not in terms of years, but in breaths. Breath control is a profound technique of experiencing and ultimately controlling the dual physical-mental Self.

How do *you* breathe?

Lie with your back flat on the floor. Lift your head slightly as you raise your knees; or, to be completely comfortable, slip a pillow beneath your head. Just breathe normally. Observe. Which parts move with your breathing? Upper chest? Stomach? Back? Does one side breathe more pronouncedly than the other? Does your neck tense as you breathe in?

Sense your abdomen and diaphragm, the latter being the large muscle separating your inner chest from your inner abdomen. The diaphragm is the workhorse of the respiratory system. It contracts and plunges down toward the stomach, creating a hollow into which air rushes. This pushes the abdominal organs down toward the pelvis, and slightly outward, so the stomach and lower back swell a little. Exhalation is a passive process: The diaphragm just lets go, relaxes to its original position, shoving the lungs back up until they have no room for all that air. As the air is expelled, the rib cage shrinks, along with the volume of the lungs.

Tension in the rib cage, back, or stomach muscles can keep the lungs from expanding to their fullest. Try some tests: As the diaphragm contracts downward, feel your lower back. Make sure those muscles and ribs are free to expand. This back breathing is very important. It means the air is rushing to the very bottom of the lungs. Now do the same with your side ribs. Are they as loose as they should be? Do they expand laterally as you inhale? Move your hands to your chest and feel it rise with each inhalation. Make sure there's no constriction in your chest. Finally, put your fingers to your collarbones, to determine whether breath is entering all the way to the top of the thorax. Do your collarbones rise as you breathe in?

Having checked yourself over, you're ready to do two favorite yoga breathing exercises, *Ha Breathing* and *The Lion:*

1. HA BREATHING. Stand with your arms at your sides. Your feet

should be at least a shoulder's width apart. The palms of your hands are turned inward.

First breathe out, voiding your lungs *completely*. Then inhale slowly through the nostrils as you lift your arms above your head. Let the upper part of your body fall forward from the hips. As you do so, you needn't utter a sound but you must mouth the word "Ha!" as though you were shouting it while simultaneously exhaling through your mouth.

Let your head and arms dangle. Be sure your neck muscles are equally relaxed. As you straighten up, lift your arms once more above your head as you slowly inhale through your nose. Then drop your arms slowly to your sides, exhaling very slowly, and return to starting position. In the beginning, repeat at least three times; gradually increase to ten times.

2. THE LION. Sit on your heels. Place your palms on your knees. Take a deep breath. Then exhale violently, stretching your jaw down in an exaggerated way and poking out your tongue as far as you can. At the same time, spread your fingers fanwise and stiffen your hands, forming claws. Freeze for a few seconds. Then relax. Repeat at least three times.

Into your exercise program and into every activity of the day, incorporate your newfound awareness of the flow of breath. Delight in its rhythm and tranquillity.

□ *USING TENSION AS A GROWTH TOOL*

It's time to insert a reminder that stress is natural enough and that tension can be useful. Your health and beauty depend upon how well you cope with and master tension. Everything we've cited and discussed so far assures us that the best antidote for nervous tension is to become physically tired.

Golden Door guest Georgiana Sheldon would like to see employers across the country set up exercise rooms where employees could work out muscular kinks and tensions.

"In my opinion, employees would feel better, work better, and enjoy their jobs more," says this vice-chairman of the Civil Service Commission. And she practices what she preaches. Even during the harrowing weeks following the Guatemalan earthquake of February 1976, when Georgiana kept office hours from six A.M. till midnight or past, being in charge of disaster relief for the State Department, she found the time for a few minutes of yoga.

Listen to another woman who uses all her senses and all her energy on the job every day. On my most recent trip to New York I stopped by the *Vogue* offices to see art director Rochelle Udell. And I kept thinking of the change in her since her first day at The Golden Door seven months before.

"Well, you know I went to The Golden Door at a time when I really needed it," she recalled.

> I'd been working quite hard. I'd been through a divorce. In a year I'd put on fifty pounds. Except for my work, everything I'd been doing was self-destructive. I couldn't see myself; I literally had padded my life with activities, and with fat, so that there wasn't any center anymore. I didn't know where I was in the middle of all that, and I didn't want to know.

She had been starved for time to be alone with herself. "In two weeks at The Golden Door," she continued,

> I had to come to terms with a number of things, including how to handle the high-pressure kind of work. We're constantly meeting deadlines against incredible odds . . .

The most efficacious tranquilizer for Rochelle turned out to be running. At first the lesson of the morning walk at The Door helped. Now, after her third visit to The Golden Door, she not only walks to work (a one-mile distance), but begins each day with a run.

> The running established a balance in my life (Energy begets Energy). I now have worked up to a minimum daily run of three miles (and a six- or eight-mile run three times a week), and every tenth day or so I don't run—my body lets me know when to stop. You learn to listen to it. That's the greatest lesson learned at The Door: "Reading one's own body."
>
> I have mirrored walls in my apartment and am not afraid to look. Deborah taught us to begin each day with a "look and see," and she insisted that I redo my kitchen so that it is visually satisfying and the gratification need not come entirely from food.
>
> But the big breakthrough was understanding that I hated regimented exercise classes and I loved sports. I now approach exercise as a way of life, running daily (and playing tennis for fun), and I reward myself with a massage once a week.

□ MASSAGE AS A REWARD

Touching is such a basic form of communication that it can do all sorts of things to untwist the emotions. Rubbing yourself down with a towel, giving yourself pats and strokes, can make all your skin's nerve ends say "thank you." But massage—being stroked artistically by an expert—makes you feel better still.

Massage is an ancient art which has been practiced by every culture. An expert can take you beyond relaxation and mere good feeling and provide you with an actual healing experience. The process is all fluidity and grace. Everything happens slowly, rhythmically, and quietly. It literally modifies your breathing. Afterward all is smooth as quiet energy surges through you.

Don't schedule a massage till you really want to take the time to unwind and be a completely passive subject. If you can't relax easily, wait until your exercise program is well under way and you're feeling smug and virtuous. When you know you've earned a special treat, it will be easier to surrender to what many people still consider a sybaritic form of relaxation.

Be a comparison shopper if you have no trusted friend to guide you in choosing a masseuse or a masseur. Select someone of the same sex who is licensed and who doesn't make you nervous. It's best at first to go through a health club or a similar institution with a spotless reputation. And you can call an established school of massage instruction, which probably will refer you to legitimate graduates near you, perhaps even to someone who will come to your home. Massage administered in private, familiar surroundings is even more devastating to the tensions. For this reason our Golden Door guests receive daily Swedish massage in their own rooms.

□ CREATIVE SLEEP

Having learned daytime relaxation, you can apply it to nighttime rest. It's possible to enhance the quality of your sleep and turn it into an effective ally of beauty and health.

If you experience sleep problems, devise a calming atmosphere before you go to bed. Be consciously involved and feel you're preparing for a renewing experience; avoid serious conversations that stir up emotions before sleep. Forget the prototype Golden Anniversary couple ascribing marital and personal longevity to their always settling any quarrel just before tucking in. Don't take the chance. Nearly every sleep researcher has found that the most common cause of restless sleep is emotional turmoil. Give yourself the opportunity to be calmed down, not riled up.

Keep a growth book at your bedside—poetry, the Bible, Marcus Aurelius, Lao-tzu—thoughts to put you into a comfortable frame of mind and lift you above petty worries and cares. The Golden Door weans away many insomniacs by providing every guest with nightstand copies of Erich Fromm's *The Art of Loving* and Paul Tillich's *The Courage to Be*.

If sleep still eludes you, the old remedy of warm milk is helpful for the very logical reason that milk contains the amino acid tryptophan, known for its mild sedative qualities. Heat the milk to hurry it into your system. Then lie down and perform some progressive-relaxation exercises, starting with one foot, next the other, working evenly upward on both sides of your body. Think of ocean water and a gentle, swelling surf; or a plangent wind streaming through deep, sweet, yielding grass; or birds rising in almost effortless flight as if someone had just touched an antigravity button; or whatever imagery brings you peace.

At some time or other everybody wakens in the middle of the night. If your mind then insists upon wandering back to daytime cares, do sit up, turn on the light, and read a bit more.

□ *DREAMS AS FRIENDS AND TEACHERS*

Since there are so many books about dreaming, this book won't go into the subject in any detail, except to say you'll probably rest better if you approach dream interpretation in the spirit of the Senoi people of Malaysia. The Senoi see their dreams as friends and teachers and are grateful for whatever comes to them in sleep. Why be upset if you can't figure out a dream, or if it casts you in a bad light? You provided the scenario, produced it, directed it and acted in it. Don't be alarmed. Whatever the story line, it involved no real action or risk; you were in no physical danger.

The wakening brings you back to reality, and a bit of creative analysis may put the dream into perspective so that you may use it as a pathway to your own inner processes. Were you an observer? Was it uphill? There are many interesting books you may wish to research which will help you to use your dreams as a teaching tool. The triggering event is almost always an event of the preceding day, often in itself of little significance, but when it reverberates with something at a deeper level it can emerge into another level of consciousness as your dream.

I'm opposed to the ten or eleven o'clock news, and invite you to involve yourself during the hour immediately preceding sleep with creative, soothing pursuits. I personally have found this hour to be best for reading philosophy, feeling a direct link with the philosophers of long ago who spent sleepless nights just to consider the mysteries of the universe, the thoughts that I imprint into my consciousness as I fall asleep.

Beware of an excess of sleep. Keep in mind that your metabolism slows down when you sleep. For that reason, over weeks, months, years, even a moderate eater can sleep herself into overweight. Also, too much sleep can make you feel sluggish and out of touch the next day. So, if you awaken feeling tired, it's usually another indication that more emphasis needs to be given to quality rather than to quantity.

After forty, you may find, as most people do, that you require less sleep every decade. Experiment. I find I do very well on six hours a night, and I love that extra hour to read, play, and do all the things I enjoy more than sleep.

☐ MEDITATION

Meditation may be vital to your survival. It well may turn out to be the best single means of avoiding future shock, of acting sensibly and selectively, and of guaranteeing your peace of mind. The time of simple activism is past. We no longer live in an orderly world where hard work and persistence and great deeds alone pay off. Nor is passivity an answer.

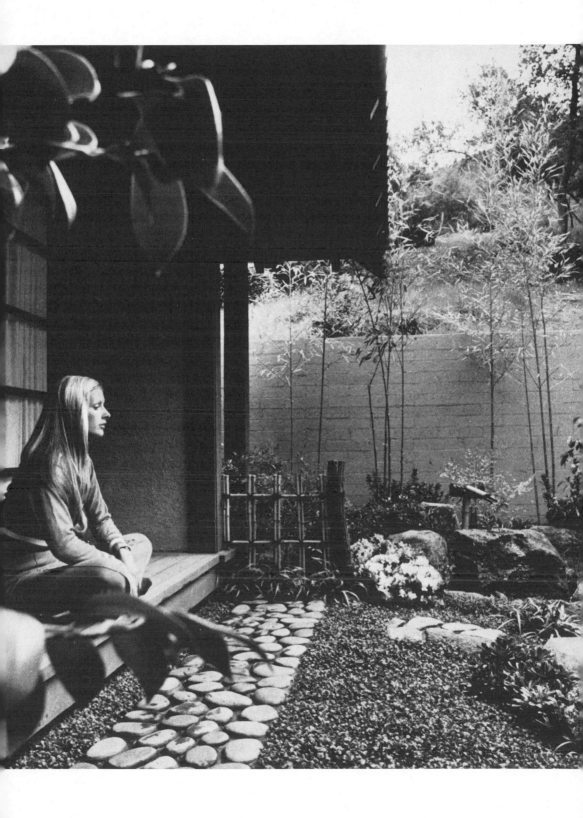

Based upon both my own experience and witnessing the changes meditation has wrought in many of my guests, I'd say this discipline helps you along the route to the journey's end of this book: learning to live for *life*.

Meditation is the flip side of the mental process of thought. It's non-thought. When you think, you're systematically involved in construction work, like a child with building blocks. But in meditation, by using a variety of techniques, you can slow down your teeming brain and let it lie fallow. Your body needs to stop and start and stop again. So does your mind.

One technique of meditation involves focusing your mind on one object, such as a vase, or the bowl in the Japanese tea ceremony. After you have sat for a time, this simple and familiar container loses its everyday aspect. It looms unfamiliar and full of unrealized potential. This is the essence of meditation: It enables you to slip outside your own mind and give your brain a half-turn, so you view yourself and the world from a new perspective, perceiving the same old things in a fresh way. Blake caught it in his insightful stanza:

> To see a world in a grain of sand,
> And heaven in a wildflower,
> Hold infinity in the palm of your hand,
> And eternity in an hour.

Meditation is not withdrawal. It's an intuitive process, as opposed to the thinking process. You need not practice meditation in a vacuum any more than you have to leave the world behind you in order to do simple thinking. Rationality *and* intuition make fine companion tools for living.

Although millions have taken up meditation of one sort or another, it is still developing as a mass phenomenon. No one knows all the forms it may assume as it penetrates our culture. I'm convinced it will enhance our health. Explore: examine the many forms of meditation until you chance upon one giving you that feeling of coming home, a recognition that *this* is the one for you. But never stop looking and learning.

Should you find one book, one system, one master apparently supplying you with all the answers to the riddle of life, then heed the Zen parable: "If you meet a Buddha on the road, slay him!" This means that you must adhere to your own path of enlightenment and accept no gurus. Preserve your own subjective view of life. To find a pat system for coping with all of the world, man, and nature would simply be a denial of living and the beginning of death—for living is the process of growth and learning.

□ DRUGS: THE TECHNOLOGY OF SENSE MANIPULATION

We don't spend much time with prohibitions, since we're much more interested in determining what you should do than bothering about what you shouldn't. It's true, though, that the use of drugs such as alcohol, tobacco, mood pills, and coffee should be minimized in any sincere health plan. Moreover, even such medications as aspirin, antacids, sedatives, and any common painkiller can prevent body dialogue. They mask and make temporarily bearable conditions which should have prompt diagnosis and affirmative action by you and your physician. Take medication only when the need is acute.

If you are a regular television watcher, you may find yourself persuaded that drugs of one kind or another are essential to *everybody's* happiness, success, and even survival. I asked a friend to monitor each of the commercial TV networks for one day. She filled pages with notes on headache pills, antacids, cold remedies, tonics, cures for the blahs, and the like. CBS led the misery parade with thirty-eight negative commercials in eleven and one-half hours; ABC was a nagging second with thirty-seven in ten hours, NBC clocked fifteen in eight hours. Your television set is telling you about three times an hour that there must be something wrong with you and that you'd better rush out and buy something for it.

Please note that I don't say these drugs should be eliminated totally. Alcohol in moderation is a pleasant and civilized way to augment a friendly occasion. At The Golden Door we occasionally use wine in our cooking and serve a glass of champagne on Saturdays to celebrate the termination of the week and the toasting of new friends. I do think a glass of white wine with friends is delightful as well as delicious; there's nothing very wrong with occasional social drinking—so long as it remains occasional. However, there is no doubt we would be better off if we eliminated all alcoholic beverages.

The time to cut back on all sorts of drug intake has arrived, not just because so many drugs are dangerous, but because all of them either lull, distort, or overly disturb your own awareness.

As one of my Golden Door friends says:

> Every time I used to think I felt great, I was under the influence of one drug or another, some kind of phony thing. And when people would tell me to try healthful food or exercise or body awareness, I'd say, "Aah, I'd pull a muscle or break my neck or something. Leave me alone."
>
> Now I want to keep forever this great feeling of being without an hallucinogen, Valium, or anything like that.

She has recognized the incomparably heightened awareness that is the first step upward in consciousness raising and is also the foundation for a lasting sense of well-being.

□ SMOKE GETS IN YOUR EYES . . .

It also gets in your skin crevices, and other people's lungs and hair.

When cigarettes were popularized at the end of the last century, young people who affected worldliness used to refer to them jocularly as "coffin nails," little guessing how appropriate that epithet might be.

I'm glad to report that social customs at last are being turned around. Regardless of statistics establishing that the habit of smoking is on the rise, particularly among the young, it's less and less socially acceptable. Grace Bechtold, my Bantam Books editor and a Golden Door guest, confirms it. "I'm not as impressed by the arguments about health, since my health is okay. What's starting to get to me very badly is that smoking is becoming more and more repulsive to a lot of people. And who wants to be repulsive? To anybody?"

Not all friction is among business acquaintances. I overheard one guest tell another, "Since I gave up smoking I've had problems with my sex life. When I kiss my wife, it's like kissing an ashtray."

Here is a theory I've intuited—there's no scientific evidence at all:

It would seem to me that each and every time one inhales tobacco smoke, the capillaries immediately affected are the ones adjacent to the nasal passages and to the brain. These thus receive a shade less of that most vital substance, oxygen. The idea is not so farfetched, since it's generally accepted that constriction of the capillaries is part of the effect of smoking. What an alarming thought, for within the brain lies our ability to live fully.

□ TIPS TO HELP YOU QUIT SMOKING

If you feel you can't quit smoking overnight—and there are millions like you—perhaps one or some or all of the following five methods will help:

1. Make it inconvenient to smoke by keeping cigarettes in relatively inaccessible places.

2. Keep a log of each cigarette you smoke; note the time and the circumstances, as well as your emotional state.

3. Write down your reasons for wanting to quit; then remind yourself frequently of all the advantages of not smoking.

4. Consciously change all the habits and circumstances associated with the times you smoke.

5. When you have gradually but methodically cut down to one pack a day, you're ready to try the drastic plunge: cold turkey.

A change of pace and place worked remarkably well for Calvin Klein, the fashion designer. In addition to three ready-to-wear collections, Calvin also designs two yearly collections for a suede-and-leather company, plus scarves, furs, and linens.

"It's normally a high-pressure business," says this three-pack-a-day man. "I work late a great deal of the time, and when we're setting up a show it's not unusual for me to work twenty-four hours without stopping."

One day he broke a promise to join friends on a trip to South America. "It was going to be one of those twenty-four-hours-a-day partying trips. I didn't need that," says Klein, who engages in meditation and the study of mind control. Instead he went to Rancho La Puerta.

I got up at six-thirty, climbed a mountain, breathed fresh air, ate healthful food, exercised, got a lot of sun and went to bed early. It was incredible! The second day, I didn't want a cigarette. And I didn't smoke again until I left after seven days. I had a sense of being healthy. I felt happy. It was the greatest.

If you really want to kick the habit, and all else fails, check the yellow pages of your telephone directory and settle on one of the many peer-group therapy organizations that have good track records because they reflect some of the A.A. philosophy: Each fellow sufferer helps the other, and even the leader/teacher at one time was a victim, too.

□ REALLY CARING
ABOUT SKIN CARE

It's fitting to close a chapter on the body and all its senses by paying tribute to your skin, which packages everything so miraculously. Treat it tenderly.

Your skin is a fantastically intricate sensory receiver and transmitter—it advertises to the outside world your inner state.

If you want perfect skin, good heredity helps. There isn't a thing that you can do about your genes. But there's plenty you can do about exercise, the food you eat, and the water you drink. Carelessness in these crucial matters shows up in the skin more quickly than anywhere else.

Your delicate facial skin is constantly subjected to external irritations. Excessive wind and sun dry it. Smog and chemical wastes assail it. Ingredients contained in your own cosmetics may be assaulting it. Add to this the skin's own debris as it sheds cells and excretes sweat and oils, and you have a bothersome combination. Dead cells, when abandoned on the skin's surface, roll up inside any tiny creases. Removing this microscopic trash from your skin is what effective cleansing is all about.

Each person has, on the average, about two square yards of skin; it varies in thickness from one-thirty-second to one-eighth of an inch, and weighs about seven pounds. Each hardworking square inch harbors nearly twenty billion cells, six hundred fifty sweat glands, over two hundred fifty sensors for heat and cold and pressure, some one hundred sebaceous glands, seventy-eight nerves, twenty blood vessels and muscles.

Skin does so much more than cover you. It helps to regulate body temperature, excrete waste materials, and keep some fluids in and others out. It provides the sensory transition between you and the rest of the world.

Even if treated reasonably well, the skin is sure to lose some elasticity because of the normal thickening that comes with age. But given superlative care, your skin can better renew itself and stay young-looking longer.

□ *CLEANSING AND CAMOMILE*

Hungary has given the world many famous international beauties and professional beauty advisors. I am told this is due to the Hungarian woman's preoccupation with facial cleansing, simplified for her by the availability of good water and the tradition of using camomile, which has been valued as a complexion safeguard for thousands of years.

Because the sensitive skin can suffer broken capillaries if rubbed harshly with a washcloth, The Golden Door suggests using a water-soluble cleansing milk (not soap, which is high in alkalinity) that is removed with delicate little Italian sponges. This removes all except eye makeup, which should be taken off with camomile extract. Remove eye makeup with pieces of absorbent cotton torn to the size of small powder puffs. Do not buy the ready-made cotton balls, since they contain chemicals. Never substitute cleansing tissue, for it contains abrasive root particles.

Camomile can be bought in any health-food store that has a line of herb teas. Brew the camomile leaves as though preparing tea (buy the loose herb leaves, not the bags). You can soak your cotton eyepads in camomile and then put them on your eyes to relieve puffiness.

After you have applied the water-soluble cleanser, you will want to remove the residue left on your face. Again, employ your cotton puffs—twenty if necessary—after wetting them with a little water, followed by a skin freshener. In buying a freshener, look for one without alcohol if your skin is dry; as much as 8 percent alcohol will be suitable for normal skin; 20 percent alcohol is ideal if your skin is oily.

It is a good idea to search your face for whiteheads during the cleansing operation. Dab at them with Q-tips dipped in skin freshener.

(Of course, when I talk about facial care, I mean your face, throat, and neckline area.)

Never cleanse your skin more than twice a day, unless you go out in the evening. Unless you have an oily complexion you need not cleanse it in the morning—you went to bed with a clean face.

In the morning, splash tepid or cool water on your face ten or fifteen times. Follow this by splashing with a skin refresher (no alcohol) to close your pores and wake you up. Camomile will befriend you in the morning, too. Spray your face with mild camomile tea, which you have refrigerated in a spray bottle. Your face will be left soothed by an oil substance in the camomile. Then apply a light moisturizing lotion as a protective base. It is also in the morning that you should apply eye cream—not at night.

Last, to arm yourself against the day, use a good covering makeup foundation. Fortunately, these are once again in fashion. Fashionable or not, they are a protection and a necessity.

Besides your daily cleansing routine, you must add weekly ones. A facial sauna is a multi-purpose cleanser, loosening dead cells, purifying clogged pores, stimulating your skin's circulation, and providing the water your face needs in order to be smooth and young-looking. Again, rely on camomile leaves. A ten-minute camomile facial sauna will benefit every type of skin. You do not have to buy a facial-sauna machine. Substitute the old-fashioned pot-a-boiling on your stove top, and make a tent over it and your head with a large towel, but do be careful to turn the heat off after water's boiling.

A mask is a weekly must as well—clay for cleansing, a gel or non-drying mask for moisturizing. If you, like most people, have a combination complexion—fairly oily on the forehead-and-nose T-zone but rather dry elsewhere—you will find it expeditious and doubly beneficial to use both types of mask at one time.

Another dividend-paying once-a-week ritual is the exfoliating mask or lotion, a gentle, invisible way to accelerate the removal of dead skin residue. It may show you that although the top layer of your skin appears dry, there is normal skin just beneath. More costly but worth considering is the rotating electric brush (of goat hair) for dusting off the shedding outer layer.

□ *HOW TO USE THE CRÈME DE LA CREAM*

You probably have already found a nourishing cream or a night cream that is compatible with your skin type. But the best beauty-care products in the world are not very good unless they are used properly. First of all, try to use one product line because the individual preparations are keyed to one another and can do their best work together. It probably will be better not to use the same cream on your forehead, which is apt to be a bit oily, that you apply to your throat, which is apt to be at least a bit dry. You might use two different preparations from the same line; another way would be to alternate two face creams from the same line. The changeover will keep your complexion stimulated enough not to become lazy.

Most people use more cream than is necessary. The skin can absorb only so much. If your skin is so dry that you feel the first thin application isn't sufficient, wait a bit and reapply. It's a good plan to cream your face after your nightly bath or shower, and then remove any excess before getting into bed. Your skin should breathe during the night.

An expert would vary some of the above advice according to the part of the world in which you live. In rain, for example, you would not need to use the richer of your two face creams. And if your home has air conditioning and/or steam heating, you will be wise to combat this drying effect by setting out several shallow bowls of water (so that the water evaporates) containing two little flowers—ideally, a Japanese flower arrangement very like those gracing each *tokonoma* at The Golden Door. This will keep the moisture in your skin.

□ *SKIN CARE FOR MEN*

You probably have heard the theory that the daily shave, which scrapes away a great many of the dead cells that cling to the face, is the reason many middle-aged men look younger than middle-aged women. But at The Golden Door we have demonstrated that men re-

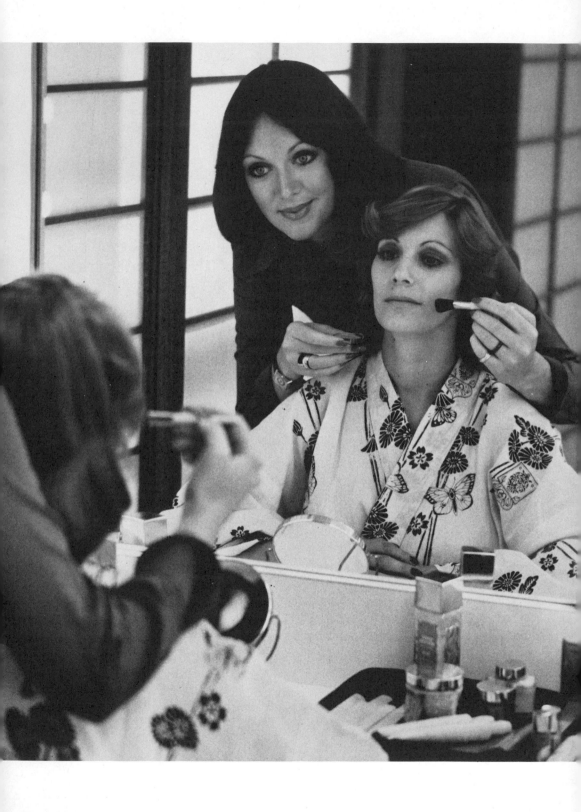

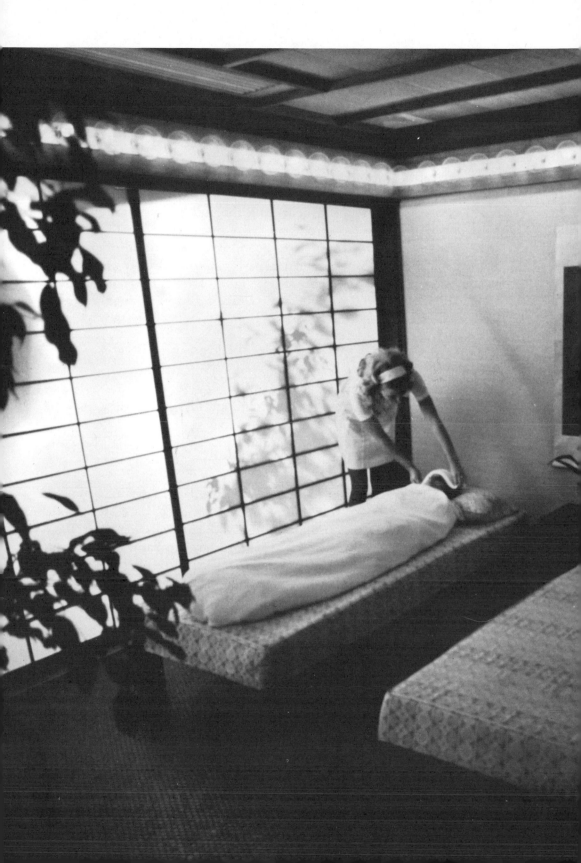

quire more assiduous cleansing than women do. That's partly because men so far have neglected their complexions and partly because men have larger facial pores and oilier skin than women. This leaves them more susceptible to blackheads.

Although a lot of men still imagine there's something unmanly about complexion care, all would benefit from the use of a good water-soluble cleansing milk at least once a week. Our male guests at The Golden Door want to feel good and look good, and their built-in prejudice against skin care vanishes as their skin becomes positively clean.

Here's one last word of skin-care wisdom for both men and women: When leaving a swimming pool, always take care to thoroughly cleanse from your face the chlorine residue.

□ WATER WORKS WONDERS

Treat your skin to the widest possible range of water pressures and temperatures. Try this refresher: a long, steamy, hot bath with your favorite herbal scent to lull you into drowsiness, followed by a sudden splash of cool water to revive you. At some point during the bath, wake up your body (not your face) with a sponge-like loofah, or substitute a rough washcloth.

A fine all-over skin-awakener for your afterbath is to slap yourself briskly but lightly over your entire body with a cold wet washcloth. Or, with your hands cupped, rain light punches on your wet body from head to foot. And when you emerge from the bath, don't always coddle your skin with a velour towel if that's your custom. Use a rough Turkish or linen towel, snapping it strongly back and forth across your legs and bottom and back until the skin there is wake-up pink.

I rely on a before-dinner swim or shower when I've had a particularly tiring day. I love the feeling of the water pouring down, washing away the day's accumulated tensions. Whenever I feel like a weary prune, water refreshes me, spruces me up, unwrinkles my senses, and perhaps gladdens the fish I once was.

□ SUN

Although recent warnings against excessive sunbathing have proliferated, it remains hard for some of us to believe anything that feels so good could do serious harm. But it does. Too much sun can cause skin cancer to develop later in life. At any stage, it ages your skin. Use common sense and don't permit temporary enjoyment of a deep tan to overrule your body's sense of what's good for it. The skin loses sensitivity as it darkens and thickens. Its ability to function diminishes. You can acquire a coat of leather if you sunbathe excessively. In the temperate zones, limit yourself to a maximum of twenty minutes of bright sunshine daily, fewer as you grow older.

Always use a sunscreen if you're in bright sunlight; if you are fair and susceptible to sunburn, use a stronger sun block on sensitive spots. Your pharmacist or cosmetician can suggest one.

□ *A I R*

During too much of your life, your skin surface is captive and unable to breathe—encapsulated within garments of various kinds. Moisture can't evaporate. Oxygen and sunlight—germ-killers supreme—can't approach the skin. This perpetual covering fosters a welcoming environment for fungi and bacteria. For half an hour or so every day, go barefoot and as nearly nude as you can.

Don't be overprotective of your skin when in the atmosphere of your bedroom. Sleep bare. Let your body be on intimate terms with the climate, the temperature, and the humidity.

There's an internal thermometer in our bodies, but like many other physical abilities, our capacity to regulate our temperature will atrophy if we don't make use of it. That is why I'm opposed to the electric blanket. It hampers your body's ability to respond to communications from your closest environment.

Whether you dress in jeans or a garment with a Bill Blass label is not important. What is important, however, is how well you fit into nature's undergarment—that exquisitely sheer original, your own body. Take care of it.

CHAPTER IV

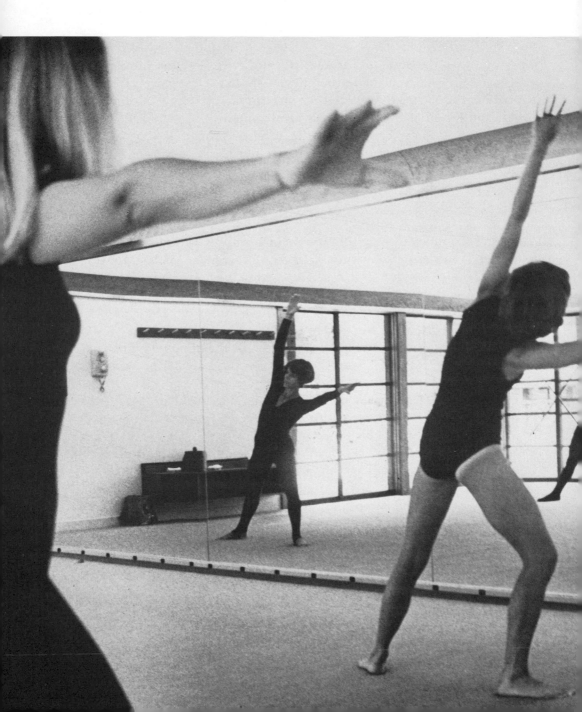

BODY AWAKENERS AND EXERCISES FOR EVERY OCCASION

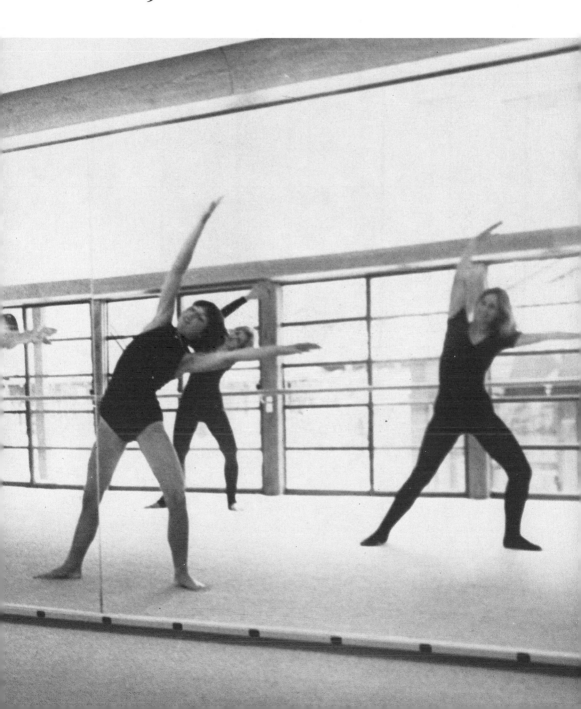

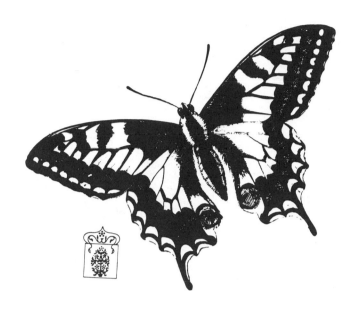

Y OU'VE PAID FOR THIS BOOK ONE-HUNDREDTH OF WHAT A WEEK
at The Golden Door costs. To make it worthwhile, you will
have to supply a missing ingredient: yourself. Yourself on the
exercise mat. Walking and jogging. Laughing and feeling
better than ever before.

All Golden Door guests arrive on Sunday, realizing full well they are
sentencing themselves to eleven-hour activity days devoted to renewing
their minds and bodies, and that much of the time will be passed at
hard labor. All ages, from teen-ager to young-at-eighty, are attracted to
this goal.

On the first morning and every day thereafter, they receive a personalized daily activity schedule. The number of class periods is always the
same, but the duration and intensity are influenced by the individual's
level of fitness and goals for the week. Here is a typical daily schedule:

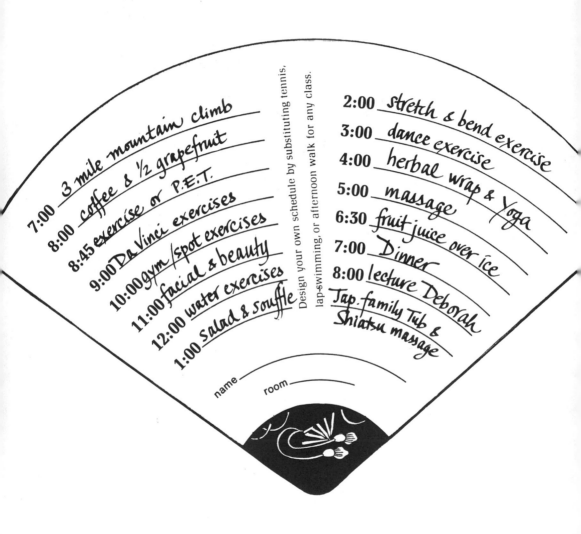

7:00 3 mile mountain climb

8:00 coffee & ½ grapefruit

8:45 exercise or P.E.T.

9:00 Da Vinci exercises

10:00 gym/spot exercises

11:00 facial & beauty

12:00 water exercises

1:00 salad & souffle

Design your own schedule by substituting tennis, lap-swimming, or afternoon walk for any class.

2:00 stretch & bend exercise

3:00 dance exercise

4:00 herbal wrap & Yoga

5:00 massage

6:30 fruit juice over ice

7:00 Dinner

8:00 lecture Deborah

Jap. family Tub & Shiatsu massage

name _____

room _____

When the guests leave The Golden Door a week later, they take with them the sum of what the instructors and I can impart to them (and what I'm striving so hard to put in this book), the encouraging example of what they have achieved in one week, the resolve to apply all this to daily living. With them go their new ABC's, which the President's Council on Physical Fitness and Sports proposes so well:

1. A regular exercise schedule
2. Supplementary physical recreation
3. Stepped-up ordinary physical activity
4. Physical activity in the day's occupation

☐ DESIGN YOUR OWN GOLDEN DOOR EXERCISE PLAN

The Golden Door judges its success by how well departing guests sustain their exercise high and integrate a regular exercise program into their own life-style. Most returnees gratify us. Some even astonish us. These are the people who use their first Golden Door week as a departure point for all sorts of self-realization.

When guests leave, they take with them a cassette which they've worked out with an instructor, that is individually designed for their own exercise program. Therefore, they are not bothered with the nagging questions of what exercises to do, in what sequence, and how many to repeat.

This is easy enough for you to do as well. Set aside a quiet hour with this book in hand, a pad and a pencil, and a full-length mirror. You also will need a cassette player, a blank thirty-minute tape, and a phonograph or a second cassette player stocked with favorite music.

Look long at yourself, nude, in the mirror. Next, imagine that you are the exercise specialist at The Golden Door about to prescribe for you which exercises you should do and the number of times you should do them. In succession, be the scriptwriter as you put the exercises in sequence; the music arranger as you select the right tempos.

That done, with script in hand and thirty minutes of happy-making music on your phonograph, talk yourself through your first exercise-program production, including warm-ups and cool-downs.

To make your first tape, start with the Golden Door Body Awakeners. You'll love being a cassette choreographer. Your tape will obviate the need to think consciously about an exercise ever again, and instead will allow you to concentrate on the feeling of movement within your body. As you become more expert you'll find you want to change your program. Just make another tape!

□ *THE GOLDEN DOOR*
   BODY AWAKENERS

This thoughtfully planned series of exercises created especially for Golden Door guests to take home with them is both isotonic and aerobic. You will recall that an isotonic exercise is one that involves rhythmic, repetitive tensing and relaxing of muscles: dancing, bicycling, walking, jogging, swimming, rowing, skipping rope, working out on a mat, and so forth. The repeated squeezing of the muscles helps the blood flow and promotes cardiovascular fitness. An aerobic exercise is one which you can continue to perform for more than a few minutes, with oxygen being supplied to the exercising muscles all during that time.

These and all exercises you will perform to music. Pick bouncy melodies with a clear, happy beat. They inspire movement. You know how a child dances when music is played. Let the child within you emerge as you too dance about your room.

Spend time selecting the music you enjoy. It should make you feel the melody in your fingertips. Each morning at The Golden Door starts off with a familiar record: "I Want to Teach the World to Sing." Whenever our guests hear it, as with a conditioned reflex, they begin to move.

Exercise mats are not essential, but they are certainly nice to have. A folded blanket will do as a substitute. The soft rug in your personal retreat is ideal.

The Golden Door often uses hula hoops, jump ropes, plastic balls (ten to twelve inches in diameter), balloons, and one-inch doweling rods approximately forty-five inches long. Yet the Body Awakeners have been designed for you to do without any equipment whatever.

Adapted from The Golden Door's famous Leonardo da Vinci exercises, the Body Awakeners consist of a twenty-minute morning program of rollicking bouncing and moving, done in specific ways designed to:

a. stretch and limber your body

b. tauten and firm body contours

c. strengthen your body

d. (most of all) make you aware of your body in everything you do

When you perform all eight Body Awakeners in order, you give every part of yourself, from your neck to your toes, a chance to participate, to confirm that it's there and trying to do its best for you.

You'll notice how very few of the eight are intended to work just a single part of your body. Since the body is an integrated system, why perform only isolated exercises for the inner thighs? The Body Awakeners are time-savers. And, as you go through all eight, you also speed up your heartbeat and breathing to a mild huff-and-puff.

If you want, you can break the Body Awakeners into individual exercises to concentrate on just one area such as waist or thighs, even though other parts of you are going to benefit at the same time. Or you may find that eight minutes of Body Awakeners, several times a day, is a magically simple formula for keeping energy high and eyes bright.

Whatever you opt for, just remember to "warm it" and "stretch it" as well as to "work it" (a sequence set by Marge Newby Samuels, who has always been invaluable in creating exercises for The Golden Door). You will notice that the Warm It and Stretch It accompaniments to each exercise are simple in the extreme and are not included in the exercise-photograph section accompanying the exercises. Now, prepare to start at an easy pace, and savor every move you make!

1 WAISTLINE CIRCLE WITH A TWIST

Benefit: To firm and slim the waist, shoulders, and upper arms.

Warm It Position: Standing, feet far apart, toes turned out; arms at sides, palms pressed against outer thighs.

Rock the upper torso from side to side, letting palms slide up and down outer thighs. Start slowly, alternate the action and increase speed.

Do twenty times.

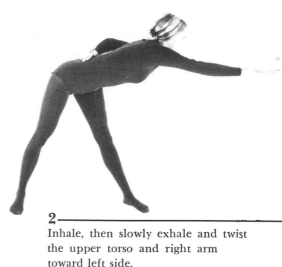

2

Inhale, then slowly exhale and twist the upper torso and right arm toward left side.

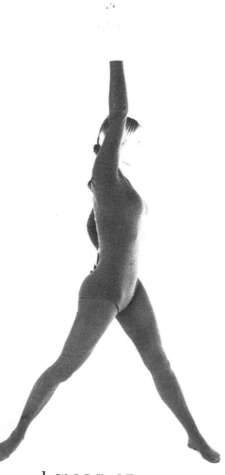

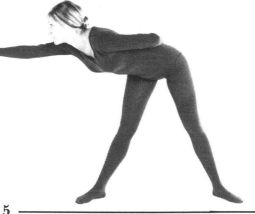

1 WORK IT

Position: Standing, feet far apart, toes turned out; left arm behind body with back of hand at belt line, right arm stretched toward ceiling.

5

Reach farther to the right and, as right arm becomes horizontal, twist torso from waist so that left shoulder pulls back.

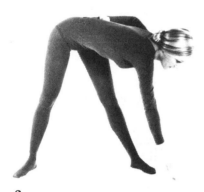

3 —————————————————
Continue the circling motion, reaching right arm down toward left toe (touching if you can)

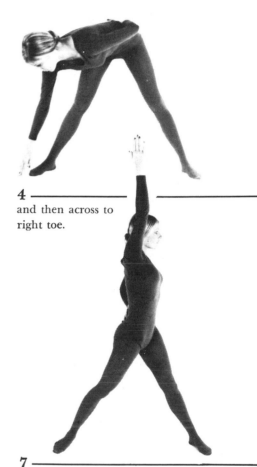

4 —————————————————
and then across to right toe.

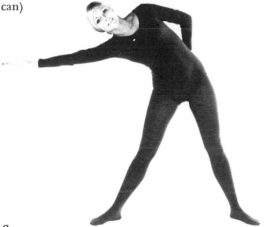

6 —————————————————
Then turn right palm upward and continue to complete the circle, on the inhale.

7 —————————————————
Finish in starting position with right arm pointed upward.

First week: Do three times, then switch direction for another three, making a total of six. Second week: As you begin to feel peppier, increase to a total of eight. Third week: Increase to ten.

Stretch It Position: Standing, feet together, fingers intertwined straight overhead, palms up.

Keeping arms straight, alternate pressing one palm at a time in a big stretch toward the ceiling.

Do ten times.

2 PITCHING HAY

Benefit: To firm the hips and inside thighs, plus arms and shoulders.

Warm It Position: Standing, feet far apart, toes turned out; hands on knees.

Bend the left knee, keeping right leg straight. Then bend the right knee, keeping left leg straight. Do ten of these left-right sets.

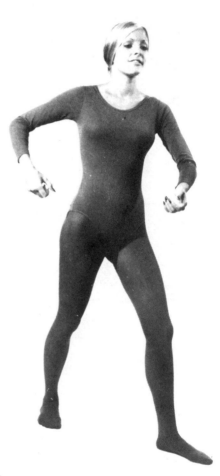

1 WORK IT

Position: Standing, with feet planted as if you are about to pitch a forkful of hay: left foot forward, hands pretending to hold the handle near your right hip. Take a deep breath.

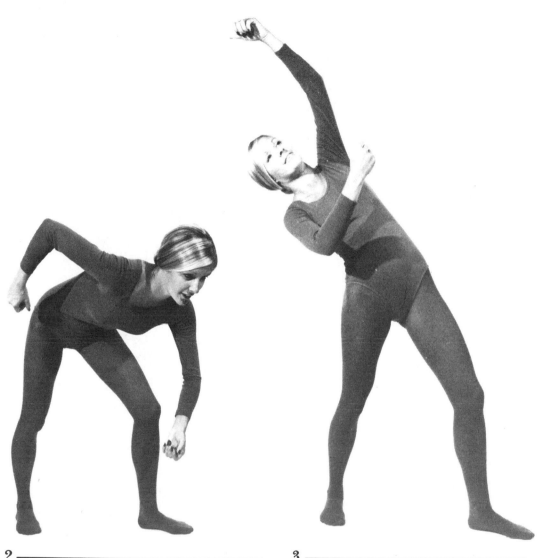

2 ————————————

Scoop both hands downward toward the forward foot, bending the forward knee as you do so, all on the exhale.

First week: Pitch five forkfuls over your right shoulder, then switch feet and pitch five over your left. Second week: seven and seven. Third week: ten and ten.

Stretch It Position: Standing, feet far apart,

3 ————————————

Then inhale, swing arms up, pitching hay over your right shoulder, imagining the make-believe hay is very heavy.

toes turned out. Keeping knees straight, bend forward from waist and let arms hang, relaxed. *Do not bounce*. Bouncing on stretched tendons will cause you pain and perhaps injury. Just hang there for a count of ten.

3 DOUBLE KNEE HUGS

Benefit: To firm the hips, thighs, and shoulder area, and to stretch the back.

Warm It Position: Standing, feet together, arms at sides.

Keeping feet together, jump lightly up and down, flexing the knees each time feet touch the floor.

Do twenty times.

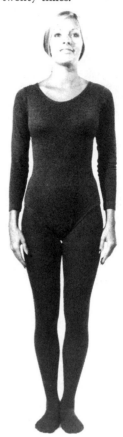

1 WORK IT
Position: Standing, feet together, arms at sides.

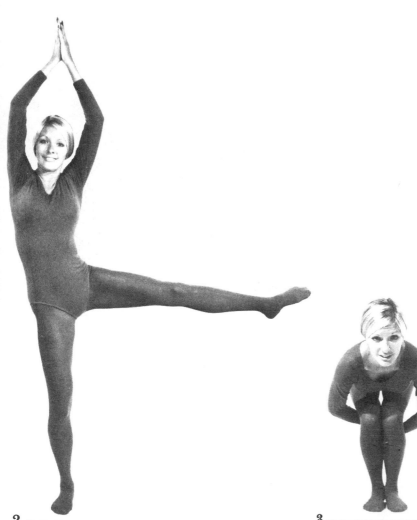

2 ———————

Take a deep breath. Clasp hands overhead while kicking left leg to left side.

3 ———————

On the exhale, bring feet together and bend knees, hugging arms behind them as far as possible while keeping heels on floor. Inhale, straightening up to starting position. Repeat all to right side.

First week: Alternating left and right, do a total of six. Second week: total of eight. Third week: total of ten.

Stretch It Position: Standing, feet far apart, toes turned out.

Take a deep breath and exhale, bending from the waist, keeping both knees as straight as possible; slide both hands down the left leg as far as you can toward left ankle. Hold there for a count of ten. Repeat to the right.

4 ROCKING HORSE

Benefit: To firm shoulder area, waist, buttocks, and thighs.

Warm It Position: Standing, feet together.

Do ten jumping jacks (clapping hands overhead as feet jump apart on the exhale; on the inhale, clapping hands to thighs as feet jump together).

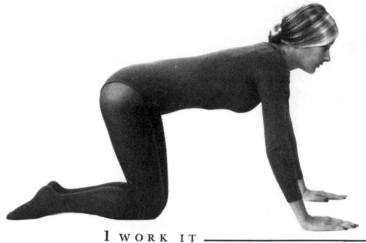

1 WORK IT
Position: On hands and knees, hands apart, knees together.

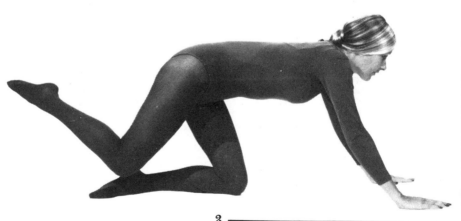

3
Slowly exhale as you stretch right leg straight back as far as possible while rocking the left hip down toward left heel.

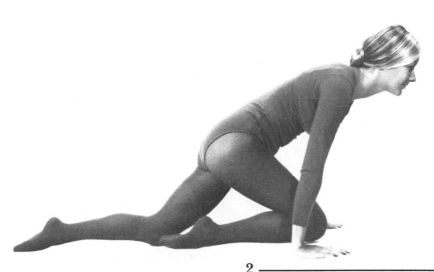

2
Take a deep breath. Bring right knee forward to touch floor between your hands.

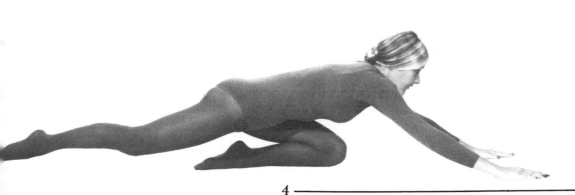

4
Touch toes of right foot to floor. Repeat, completing the full set of eight with right leg before switching to left leg.

First week: Five with the right, five with the left (total of ten). Second week: total of fourteen. Third week: total of twenty.

Stretch It Position: On hands and knees, hands apart, knees together. Rock hips back to rest on both heels. Stretch arms forward, palms down, and touch forehead to floor. Rest in this position for count of ten.

5 EXTENDED LEG CIRCLES

Benefit: To firm the hips.

Warm It Position: On hands and knees, hands apart, knees together.

Without moving hands, and keeping knees in place, lower hips to right side, then to left. (One knee will rise off the floor when you do this.)

Do five, each side.

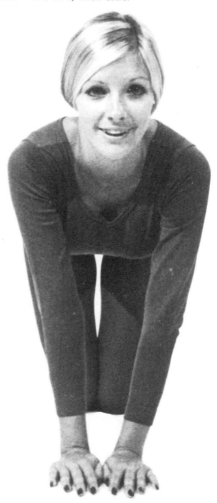

1 WORK IT
Position: On hands and knees, hands apart, knees together.

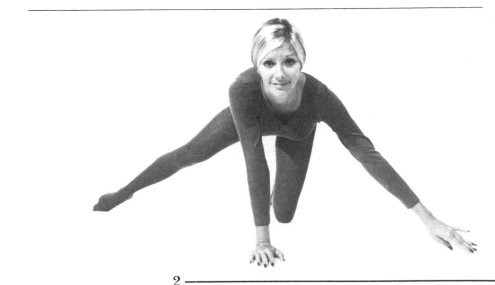

2

Move your hands slightly to the left to counterbalance the motion coming next. Extend right leg out to right side, raising foot off floor.

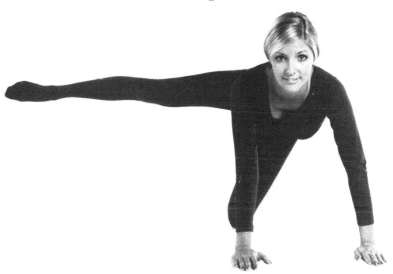

3

Keeping extended right leg straight, move it from hip so that foot describes a one-foot circle. Do this three times with a forward motion of right leg, three times backward. Then extend the leg straight back and repeat circle-making, three to the right and three to the left. Then repeat all with the left leg.

First week: Repeat the entire exercise three times. Second week: repeat four times. Third week: Repeat five times.

Stretch It Position: Lying on your back, Pull knees up to chest; clasp arms around them. Rest in this position for count of ten.

6 FALL-BACK TWISTS

Benefit: To firm waistline, pectorals, shoulder area, arms, and legs.

Warm It Position: Sitting, feet apart, legs straight.

Clasp hands in front of chest, elbows out and shoulder-high. Twist upper torso as far as it will go to right, then as far as possible to left.

Do ten times to each side, alternating.

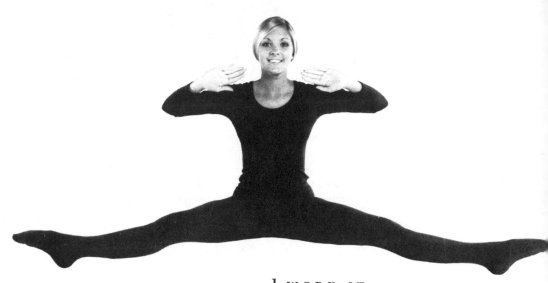

1 WORK IT
Position: Sitting, feet far apart, legs straight, hands held shoulder-high (elbows bent, palms out).

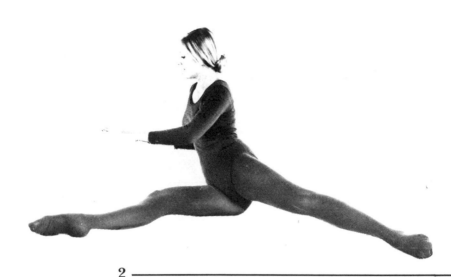

2 ───

Roll over on right hip, placing palms on floor, and lower chin to floor.

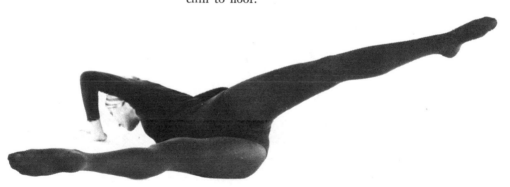

3 ───

At the same time, raise left leg toward the back (not straight up to the side). Return to starting position and reverse all to left side.

First week: Do three to each side. Second week: four to each side. Third week: five to each side.

Stretch It Position: Sitting, feet apart, legs straight.

Lean forward, sliding the right hand down the right leg as far as possible, the left hand likewise down the left leg. Grasp when you have bent as far as you can. Hold for a count of ten.

7 CROSSOVER SIT-UPS

Benefit: To firm everything from stomach up, and to stretch the legs.

Warm It Position: Sitting, feet together, legs bent, hands behind you, palms on floor.

Keeping knees together, rock them from left to right, touching a knee to floor with each rock. Do five to each side, alternating.

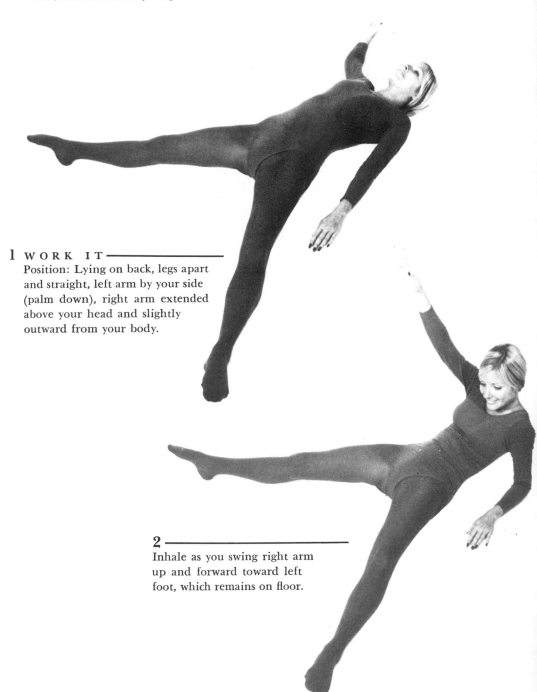

1 WORK IT

Position: Lying on back, legs apart and straight, left arm by your side (palm down), right arm extended above your head and slightly outward from your body.

2

Inhale as you swing right arm up and forward toward left foot, which remains on floor.

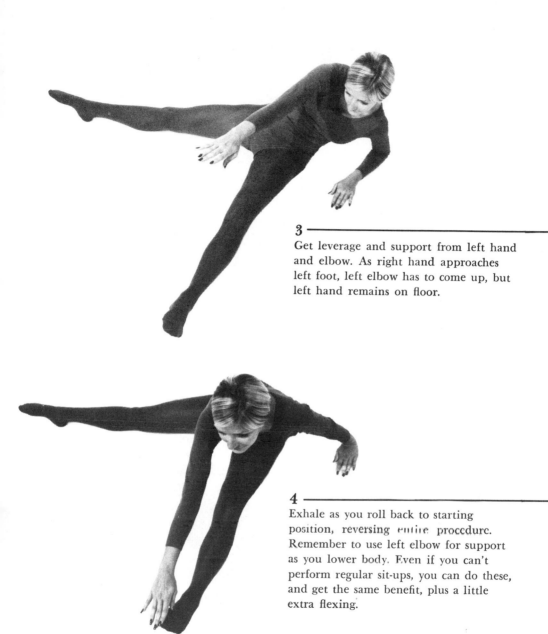

3

Get leverage and support from left hand and elbow. As right hand approaches left foot, left elbow has to come up, but left hand remains on floor.

4

Exhale as you roll back to starting position, reversing entire procedure. Remember to use left elbow for support as you lower body. Even if you can't perform regular sit-ups, you can do these, and get the same benefit, plus a little extra flexing.

Repeat, completing a full set with right arm before switching to left. First week: Do three from each side. Second week: four from each side. Third week: five from each side.

Stretch It Position: Sitting, legs together and straight.

Reach hands toward ankles, grasp legs when you've gone as far as you can bend. Hold for count of ten.

8 THE PUMP

Benefit: To firm the abdomen, upper arms, and shoulder area.

Warm It Position: Lying down on your back.

Pull knees to chest, clasp arms around them. Lift head toward knees. Roll back and forth on small of back, ten times.

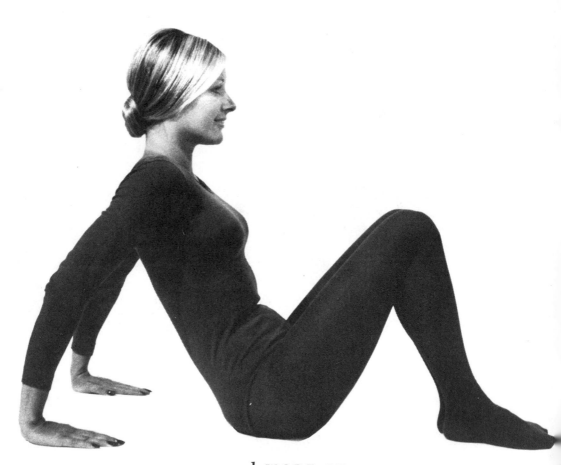

1 WORK IT
Position: Sitting, legs together and bent, hands behind you, palms facing back, fingertips to floor.

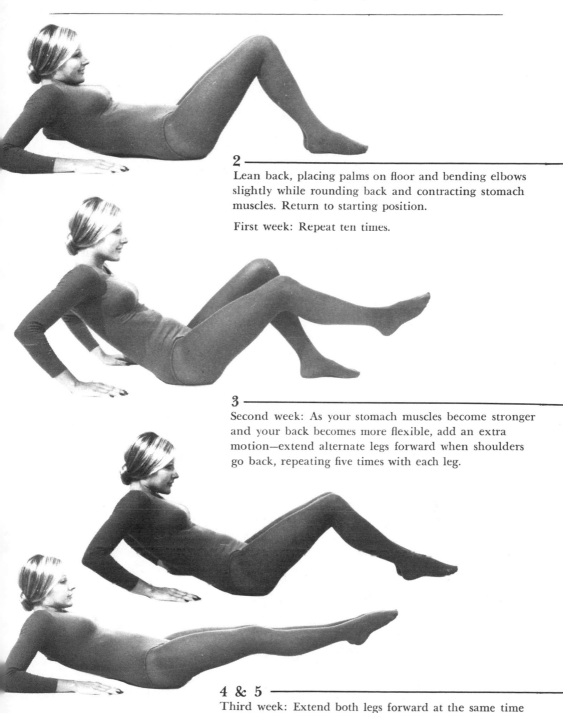

2

Lean back, placing palms on floor and bending elbows slightly while rounding back and contracting stomach muscles. Return to starting position.

First week: Repeat ten times.

3

Second week: As your stomach muscles become stronger and your back becomes more flexible, add an extra motion—extend alternate legs forward when shoulders go back, repeating five times with each leg.

4 & 5

Third week: Extend both legs forward at the same time when shoulders go back, repeating ten times.

Stretch It Position: Sitting, feet together, legs bent, hands behind you, palms down.

Lift hips as high as possible, making a "bridge."

□ OFFICE EXERCISES

The idea of little groups of exercises to be done while you take a moment or two from a frantic eight hours is not new. In my file I even have a small, undated booklet titled "Exec's-ercises" and published by the Y.M.C.A. Some of the suggestions in it are very worthwhile. For example: pull in your abdomen whenever the telephone rings, hold while speaking but do *not* hold your breath; or spend a day not using your arms whenever you stand up or sit down. The amusing cartoon figure is that of a much older-looking executive than we are accustomed to seeing today, indicating key men have improved their breed by heeding this and other good advice.

Here is some updated advice for men and women.

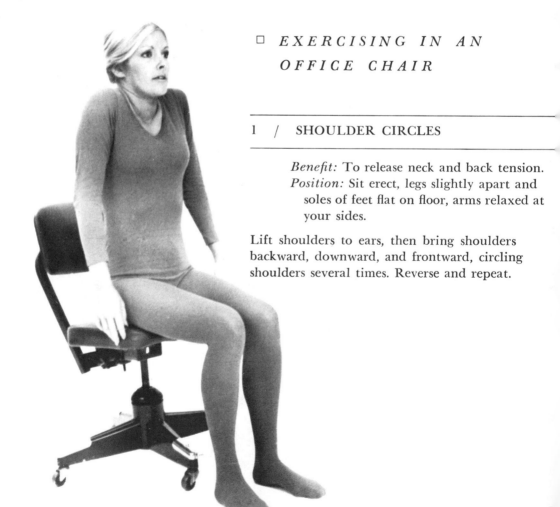

□ *EXERCISING IN AN OFFICE CHAIR*

1 / SHOULDER CIRCLES

Benefit: To release neck and back tension.
Position: Sit erect, legs slightly apart and soles of feet flat on floor, arms relaxed at your sides.

Lift shoulders to ears, then bring shoulders backward, downward, and frontward, circling shoulders several times. Reverse and repeat.

2 / STRETCH TO CEILING

Benefit: To stretch upper torso.
Position: Sit erect, legs well apart.

Raise both arms overhead and stretch toward
ceiling, reaching high, first with the right arm and
then with the left. Alternate.

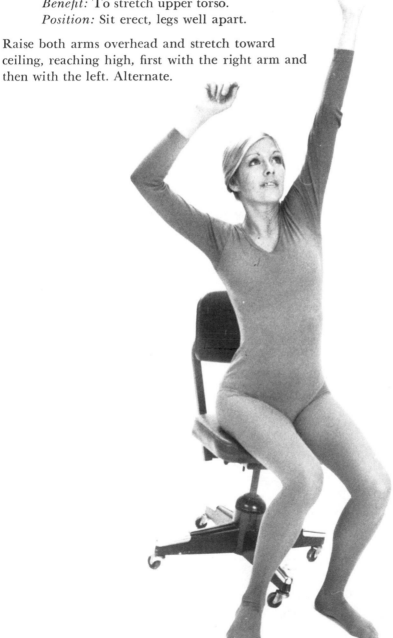

3 / SHAKE TO FLOOR

Benefit: To increase circulation in the brain
and relieve stress in the back muscles.
Position: Sit with legs wide apart.

Let head and relaxed arms drop between knees,
hands dangling on floor. Hold for several seconds.

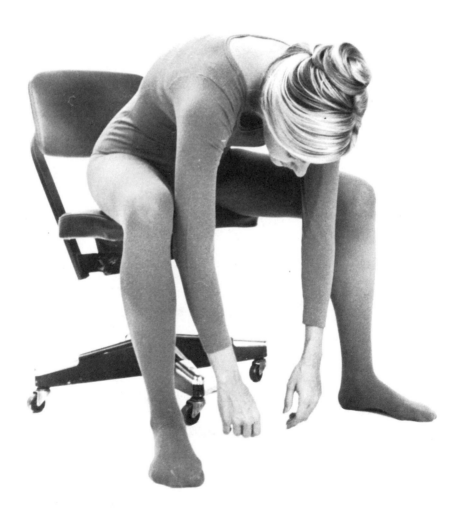

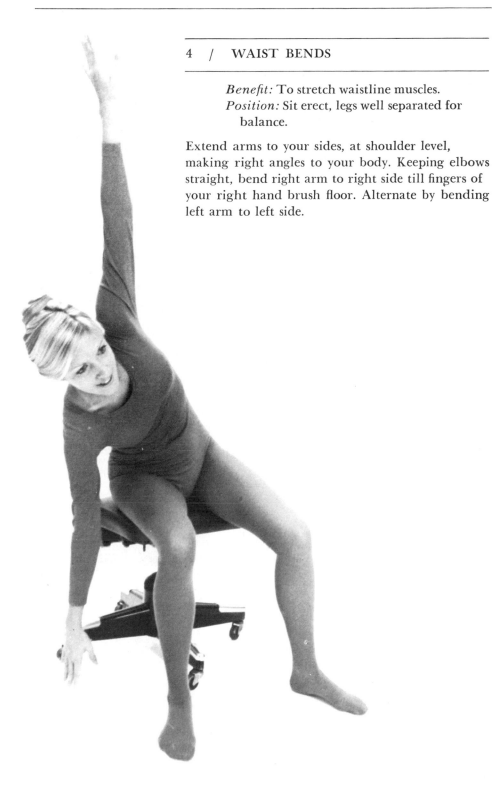

4 / WAIST BENDS

Benefit: To stretch waistline muscles.
Position: Sit erect, legs well separated for balance.

Extend arms to your sides, at shoulder level, making right angles to your body. Keeping elbows straight, bend right arm to right side till fingers of your right hand brush floor. Alternate by bending left arm to left side.

5 / KNEE HUGS

Benefit: To mobilize knee and hip joints
after long hours of sitting.
Position: Sit erect with legs slightly apart.

Clasp hands below your right knee, literally picking
up your knee and lifting it to your chest. Hug it
close. Lower your right leg to floor as you continue
to control descent with clasped hands. Alternate
with your left leg.

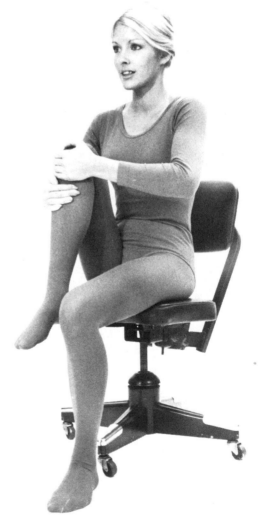

6 / TUCK AND EXTEND

Benefit: To firm flabby abdominal muscles.
Position: Sit erect, legs together.

Grasp back of chair seat. Slowly pull knees to chest
and hold for three seconds. Now extend and
straighten both legs, keeping knees tight as you
drop legs till feet touch floor.

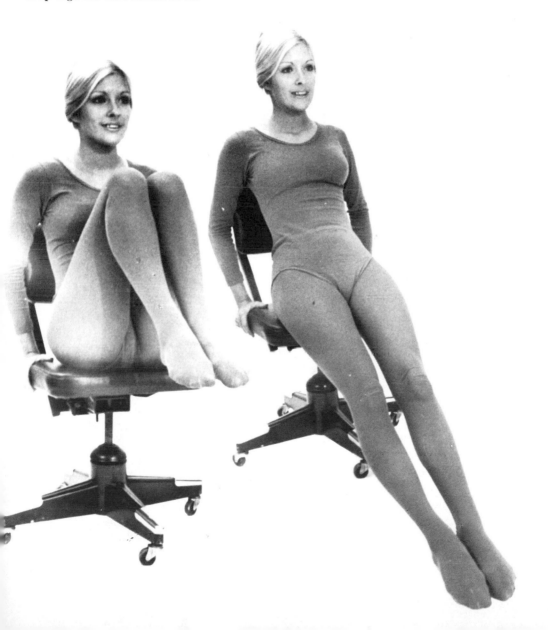

7 / CRISSCROSS

Benefit: To tone abdomen and waistline.
Position: Sit erect, legs together.

Clasp hands behind head. Lift right knee to chest
while you twist to touch left elbow to raised knee.
Drop right leg, returning right foot to floor.
Alternate with left knee and right elbow.

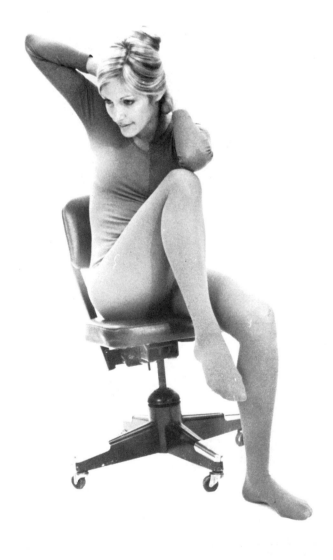

8 / BODY LIFT

Benefit: To strengthen arms and abdomen.
Position: Sit erect with legs together.

Grasp sides of your chair seat so you're sure you will be well balanced, then lift your body off chair, still keeping knees together. Hold for three seconds. Slowly drop back into sitting position.

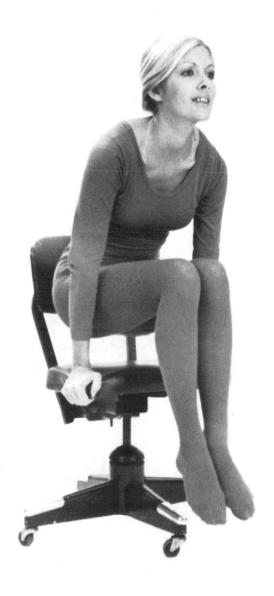

9 / WIGGLE

Benefit: To stimulate intestinal action and
tone stomach.

Position: Sit erect with legs slightly apart.
You must be well toward the back of your
chair seat.

Clasp hands behind your head. Lift right hip and
move it forward. Next, inch forward with left hip.
Continue to alternate hip movements till you
have wiggled to the front edge of your chair. Then
wiggle backward to starting position.

10 / SIDE BENDS

> *Benefit:* To stretch waistline.
> *Position:* Sit erect with legs wide apart.

Place your hands on your hips. Keep your back straight as you bend first to your right side and then to your left.

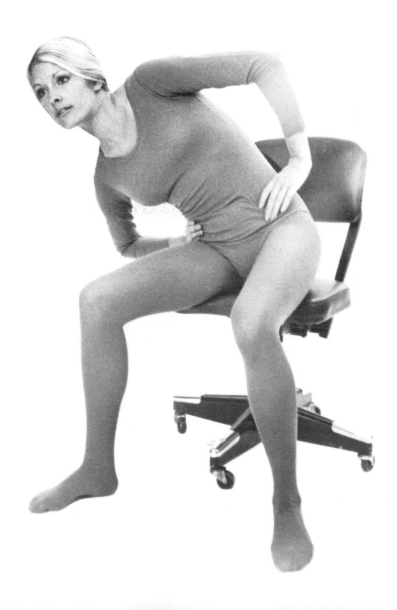

☐ BE KIND TO YOUR BACK
(PRE-EXERCISE EXERCISES)

It is said that 80 percent of the back trouble in the United States is caused by lack of exercise. Back weakness is not confined to the old. If you've been inactive, your back may have grown weaker than you suspect.

To eliminate early-week soreness in the back and other parts of the body, The Golden Door sends its prospective guests a set of conditioners and back strengtheners to practice before checking in. Then, at the outset of the new guest's first week, a class is held to help ensure that guests do not strain their backs through overdoing or lack of caution.

☐ *PRE-EXERCISE CONDITIONERS*
AND BACK STRENGTHENERS

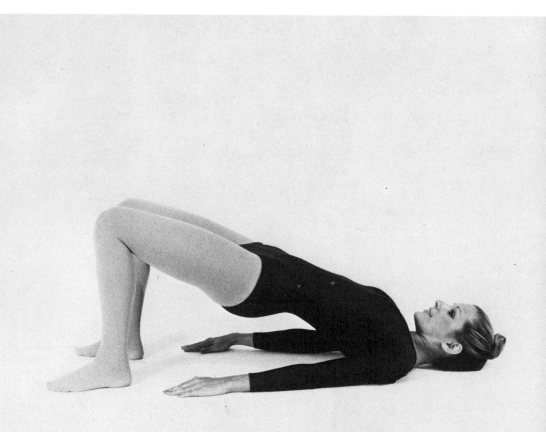

1) **Pelvic Thrust**

Position: Lying on back, hands by hips; knees bent and soles of feet on floor, twelve inches apart.

Lift pelvis slowly toward ceiling as you tighten buttocks and back muscles. Hold ten seconds, then slowly roll back down into original position; feel each vertebra touch the floor.

Repeat four times. Then repeat variation: Do with arms stretched overhead on floor, hands touching floor. Inhale on lift, exhale on roll-down.

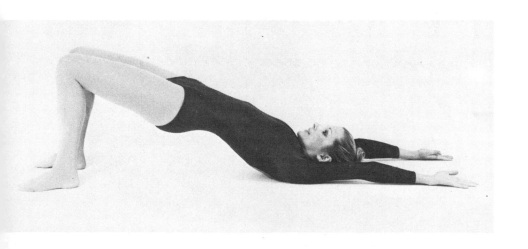

2) Knee Lift

Position: Lying on back, knees bent and soles of feet on floor; arms stretched out at sides.

Press lower back into floor as you keep knees bent and lift knees to chest. Wrap arms around knees and pull them into chest. Hold ten seconds. Relax. Exhale as head lifts and leg goes forward, inhale as head relaxes and leg pushes back.

Repeat four times.

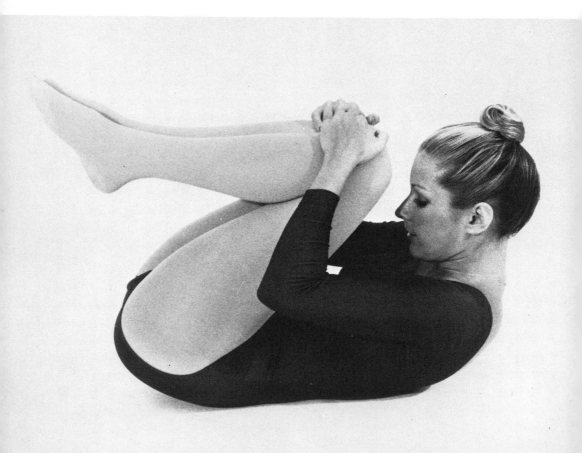

3) Torso Twist

Position: Lying on right side, bottom (right) leg bent and left leg straight; both arms stretched out to the right side, the right held slightly above the left.

Keeping left leg straight, lift it slightly off floor. Then extend left leg forward as left shoulder and arm roll back as far as they will go toward floor. Exhale as leg goes forward, inhale as leg goes back again. (As left leg goes forward, left arm, shoulder, and back will all press toward floor.) Hold ten seconds. Reverse direction, rolling left shoulder and arm forward as you move left leg backward; hold for ten seconds.

Repeat the set twice; switch to left side and perform three sets.

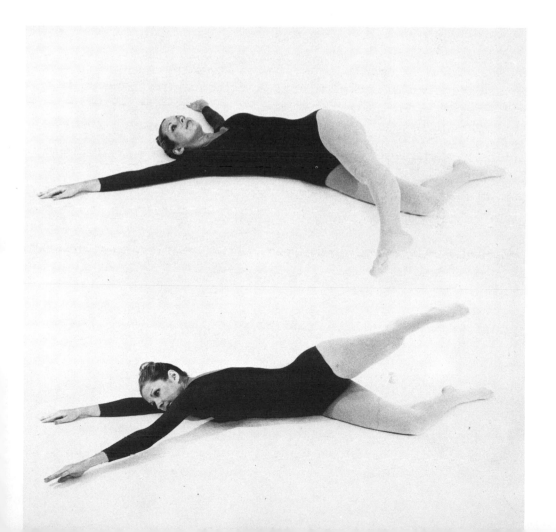

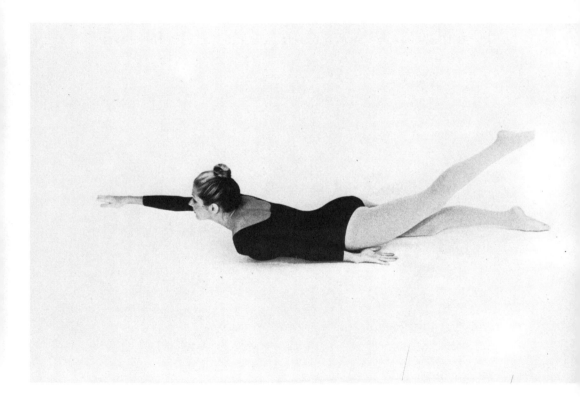

4) Back Lift

Position: Lying on stomach, legs together. Right arm is outstretched on floor above head, left arm is at side; elbows are straight.

Lift right arm, left leg, and your head at the same time. Hold ten seconds. Inhale on the lift, exhale on release.

Repeat three times, then alternate in reverse position, also three times.

5) Kitten Curl

Position: Lying on back, knees bent, soles of feet on floor; arms at sides.

Press lower back into floor. Lift knees up to chest, place hands behind knees, and straighten legs. Then lift head to knees. Hold ten seconds. Inhale on lift.

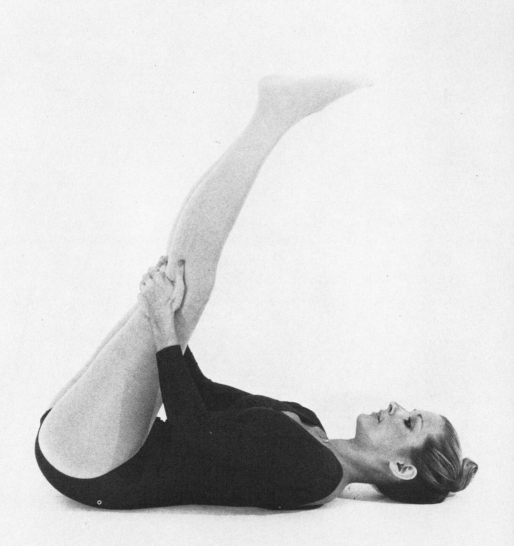

Exhale as you relax and return to original position. Repeat four times.

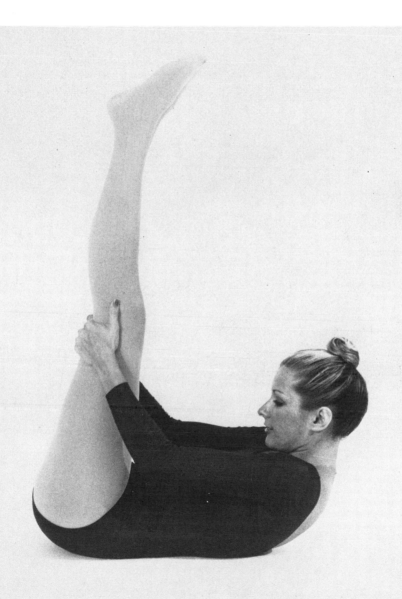

6) Wing Flap

Position: Lying on stomach, legs together. Head rests on floor, chin
   forward; palms of hands on each side of spine at midback. Elbows
   are relaxed.

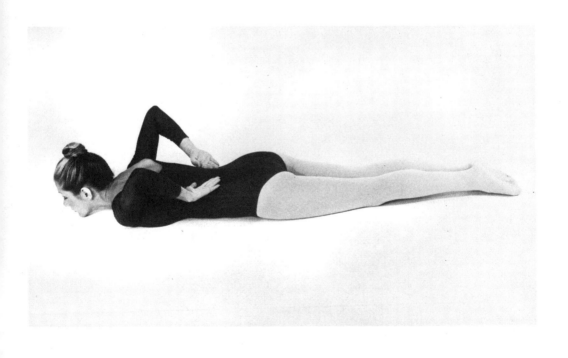

Lift elbows in back; hold five seconds. Then lift head and chest (try to relax buttocks and legs). Hold ten seconds. Inhale on the lift, exhale upon release.

Repeat four times.

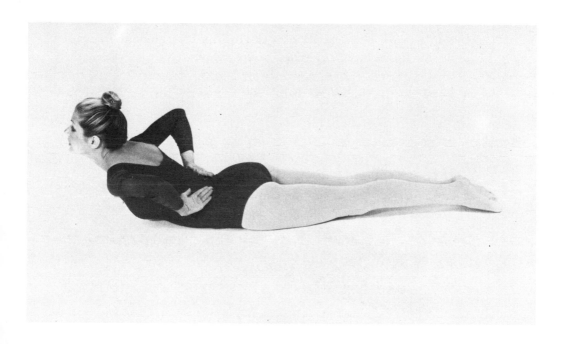

7) Prayer Position

Get down on the floor; relax your feet and sit back on your heels. Bend forward, chest to knees, stretch arms straight out in front of body, on floor. Hold for relaxation.

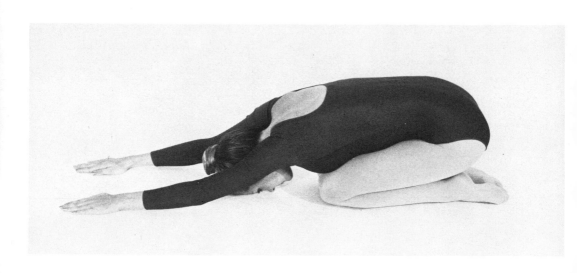

□ *SIX EXERCISE DO'S*

Remember these six prudent rules for your daily exercise:

1. DO SET ASIDE A DEFINITE TIME DAILY, MONDAY THROUGH FRIDAY. Remember, you can't store the benefits of regular exercise. If you become fit and then cut back to exercising only once a week, you will automatically drop halfway back to your original unconditioned level before ten weeks have passed. And, if you stop completely, within five weeks you'll lose all your gains.

Remember the value of locked-in exercise time. When my husband goes to our front door at seven-thirty A.M., I go with him. Each of us drives away: he to his office practice, I to the park for my rain-or-shine walking and jogging. When the children were small, I varied this by wearing my jogging suit when I drove them to school and heading for the park as soon as I dropped them off.

2. WARM UP SLOWLY.   In any exercise session, provide yourself with a few minutes of warm-ups and stretch-outs. Remember how you once warmed up your car for several minutes before you drove off, to make sure the oil lubricated all the parts? A proper warm-up helps ward off injuries by allowing the synovial fluid to lubricate each joint. Do some systematic and moderate bending and stretching.

3. BE SURE YOUR BACK IS READY, TOO.   If ever you have been plagued by lower-back pain, do begin with the special back conditioners and strengtheners (pages 130–140).

4. INCREASE YOUR LEVEL OF EXERTION.   Recognize that your respiratory/circulatory system is pleading with you daily to pay your dues to your heart by sustained exercise of at least thirty minutes' duration. Afterward, if you so desire, you can zero in on movements for reshaping, slimming down, building up, and otherwise sculpting your ideal form. (See Body Awakeners, pages 102–129.)

5. As your fitness level increases and the urge to do more becomes irresistible, alternate mat exercises with jumping rope. There are few exercises more timesaving and more satisfying.

6. COOL DOWN SLOWLY.   The body, and the heart especially, will protest as much about abrupt, brutal transitions at the end of an exercise period as at the beginning. Stopping suddenly when you have been

working out vigorously is just not sensible. Think of the runners in the Olympics, or the horses at the races. They continue to run even after they have ended the race, until their breathing has slowed to a normal rate. Also, it is unwise to conclude any workout with mat exercises that have you down on the floor—get on your feet for the finale!

You may wish to know the general level of your heart and circulatory health. And if you're over forty or have any family history of heart dysfunction, I beg you to consult your physician for advice before you take on any rigorous exercise program.

In this regard, a great guide and one I recommend to all Golden Door guests is *Beyond Diet—Exercise Your Way to Fitness and Heart Health* by Dr. Lenore R. Zohman. Developed in conjunction with the American Heart Association and the President's Council on Physical Fitness and Sports, this report may be obtained by sending ten cents for each copy to Consumer Service, Best Foods, A Division of CPC International, Inc., RFD 2, Box 373, Coventry, Conn. 06238.

□ *THREE BASIC EXERCISE DON'TS*

1. DON'T HURRY YOUR BODY. Imagine that you're a gardener. Like a plant, your body is a living organism with certain natural cycles which simply cannot be speeded up. A seed takes its own time about germinating and growing while you provide the best possible environment and tender care (which includes one irreplaceable ingredient: patience).

2. DON'T BE CONNED BY MOTOR-DRIVEN MACHINERY. When The Golden Door opened in 1959 its gym was agleam with expensive chrome muscle-toners, rollers, and other electric gadgets. I soon threw out all but the Exercycles. Motorized gadgets perpetuate the idle dream that somehow you can have your exercise done for you. Not so. Only you can make your heart pump as strongly as it wants to and should. Physical fitness is something you must get for yourself. And why not, when you are the primary beneficiary?

3. DON'T EXERCISE WHILE HATING IT. Suppose a friend has suffered an illness causing you to fear for your own level of health. Well, that's not a valid reason to start exercising. Negative motivations won't last. Besides, if you exercise with inner tension, rigidity, or anger, every

movement becomes tiring. That's because you're working against your total self instead of for yourself.

☐ ELEVEN ABSOLUTE EXERCISE TABOOS

1. Do not overdo.
2. Do not use isometric-type exercises exclusively. When you do isometric exercises, the blood vessels are contracted by extreme squeezing, inhibiting the flow of blood instead of expanding it. It is only through exercises that aid the flow of blood through the heart and large skeletal muscles that significantly improved cardio-vascular fitness is achieved.
3. Do not begin fast-action movement before fully stretching out and warming up.
4. Do not execute *full* deep knee bends if you are unused to them or unused to exercise generally. Until you achieve much flexibility and are proof against kneecap trouble, make it a rule that hips should never be brought lower than the knees.
5. Do not perform hyperextension of the back (backward and forward movements of the torso without flexing the knees). For instance, keep your knees bent when doing sit-ups.
6. Do not bounce tightly on taut ligaments as you stretch them. (A loose, rhythmic action, however, is great because it is a muscular action.)
7. Never bounce on a stretched tendon; a sustained stretch of a tendon is best.
8. Avoid excessive repetition (overworking a muscle by doing the same exercise or similar ones over and over). Exercise must flow from one movement into another, from head to foot or vice versa. If you remember that the entire body requires movement, you will not overdo on any one body part.
9. Do not lie on your back and lift straight legs without also raising your head. Or, if you are lying on your back with your head on the floor, flex your knees as you lift your legs.

10.   Don't conclude an exercise without a *moving* cool-down period—
       one which allows your pulse to return to its normal rate.
11.   Don't forget to breathe. This may sound foolish. But I have seen
       many, many people hold their breath while doing strenuous exer-
       cise. Don't perform any exercise without matching it to the normal
       breathing movements of the lungs. Generally, you should be di-
       rected to breathe in when you move upward, and to breathe out
       when you move downward.

It's apparent that a goodly number of these rules are designed to
protect the lower back of the middle-aged adult, and with excellent
reason. Because of lower-back problems, over $1.2 billion is paid out
annually by business and industry in workmen's compensation (but
seldom because of incorrect exercising, since most of the victims of
whom we speak made the error of taking no exercise at all—see page
130).

You can find the basic rules of back care and exercise in *Care of the
Back,* a twenty-four-page pamphlet published by J. B. Lippincott; you
can pick up the booklet in most orthopedists' offices.

□ POOL EXERCISING

As far as I know, Rancho La Puerta and The Golden Door were the
first major resorts to rely on water exercises and on water volleyball—
both superior forms of exercise, since you always are working against
the resistance of the water. You'll know how popular they are if ever
you come within a half-block of one of these classes and hear the bois-
terous, happy noise of the participants.

Swimming and water exercises are considered the most effective exercise for two reasons: 1) they provide a workout for the cardiovascular/
respiratory system; and 2) any movement underwater, because of the
resistance of the water, will build up the skeletal muscles faster than the
same movement done in air.

If you have access to any pool, outdoor or indoor, take advantage of
it. Many towns in this country have a pool available for public use; if
there is one near you, I can't urge you enough to make it a regular stop.

□ *GOLDEN DOOR POOL EXERCISES*

1) **Jumping Jack Cossack**

Benefit: Inner and outer thighs.

Position: Facing wall of pool. Hands in front of you, grasping pool coping; feet together.

Perform three small jumps in place. On fourth jump, go quite high,
splitting legs apart sideways, then landing with feet together. This
is a five-beat rhythm: Jump (*slow*), jump (*slow*), jump (*slow*), open
(*quick*), close (*quick*).

Variation: As you split legs apart on count number four, right leg goes
forward and left leg goes back (instead of sideways). Alternate.

Variation: When you have perfected the first two versions, then do without the aid of the pool's coping. Instead, stand in the middle of
the pool and fold arms Cossack-style as you follow the above
directions.

Begin with a set of four each and increase to eight.

2) **Water Snake Dance**

Benefit: Waist and arms.

Position: Facing wall of pool at arm's length; elbows straight and hands
grasping pool coping; feet together (make sure heels are on bottom
of pool). Throughout movement your body remains parallel to wall.

Make four full rotations to right side, four to left: You must avoid
twisting torso from side to side as you rotate your hips in a circle.
Continue with three full rotations to right, three to left; two to
right, two to left; one rotation to right, one to left—by this time,
you're really feeling the resistance of the water.

3) **Wall to Wall**

Benefit: The entire body.

Position: Standing, facing wall of pool, feet together. Hands holding onto
coping, which is arm's length away.

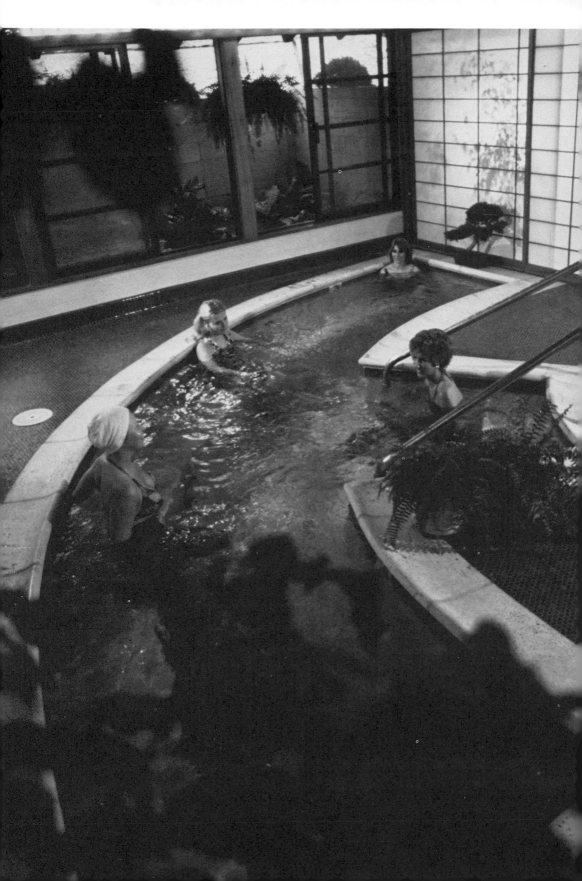

Raise right leg to right side, touching toes to pool wall as you keep right knee straight. As you lean your torso forward, still keeping knee straight and leg high, swing this right leg around in back of you and continue it around in back till your toes touch pool wall on the other side. Bring right leg back to right wall, still keeping the leg as high as possible—as if you were erasing the previous right-to-left movement.

Four times, then reverse and use left leg.

4) Writing in Water

Benefit: Waist, hips, backs of thighs, tummy.

Position: Back to wall of pool, arms extended at sides, at shoulder level, and resting on pool coping. Right foot, toes pointed, is on bottom of pool in front of you; right knee is straight.

With an imaginary piece of chalk between your right toes, and keeping right knee straight, pretend there is a blackboard sitting in the pool before you, and draw a "V" by raising right leg high toward right side, returning right foot to bottom and then immediately raising right leg toward the left, where it forms a 45° angle against your body. Return to starting position.

Alternate with left leg.

Variation: Draw a "W" by raising right leg toward right side, returning right foot to starting position, raising right leg in front of you, returning right foot to bottom of pool in front of left foot, raising right leg to left side. Return to starting position.

Alternate with left leg.

Variation: Draw a figure "8." Alternate with left leg.

5) Cut the Water

Benefit: Stomach, arms, legs.

Position: Left side is toward wall of pool. Right arm, elbow bent, is crossed over in front of you and hand grasps pool coping. Palm of left hand is pressed against the pool wall, about six inches below right hand; left elbow straight.

Stretch body to its fullest extension, toward center of pool, just as though you were lying on your left side. Scissor legs forward and back, keeping knees straight; perform scissors motion slowly and continue to stretch to fullest extension.

Do ten times. Then roll over to right side, reverse hand position, and repeat all.

6) Heave Ho

Benefit: Stomach, backs of thighs, and buttocks.

Position: Left side toward wall of pool, left hand grasping pool coping; right leg extended forward at hip height with straight knee, and parallel to water surface; right arm extended back with straight elbow.

Lean your body as far backward as possible. Then bring right arm and right leg down into the water; lean forward as you stretch the right arm forward and the right leg back. (Your knees and elbows remain straight.)

Keep repeating, with a rocking motion of the torso, ten times. Alternate to right side.

7) Waistline Wigwag

Benefit: Arms, bust, thighs, waist.

Position: Standing in center of pool, feet wide apart, knees bent, back straight. Arms straight out at sides, at right angles to body. Be certain your shoulders and arms are underwater.

Twist upper torso to right side, making sure arms keep their position and do not move either forward or back. Twist torso back to center position and then twist torso to left.

Repeat twenty times.

Variation: For upper back and midriff. Back, feet, and legs in same position; hands clasped in front of body; arms outstretched with straight elbows. Arms and shoulders are underwater.

Pivot upper torso from side to side, making sure arms keep their position and do not move either forward or back.

Variation: For arms and back of waist. Feet position same. Shoulders and arms underwater. Knees straight. Bending slightly forward from waist, lower your arms and practice golf swings underwater.

Variation: For back of arms, pectorals. In golf-swing position, bent over with clasped hands and straight knees, contract your stomach muscles as you unclasp your hands and bring them to the top of the water. Return to starting position, and clasp hands again.

Note: Repeat all variations twenty times.

8) Balinese Water Dance

Benefit: Waist and arms.

Position: Walking position. Shoulders and arms must be underwater. Right arm is outstretched at side, at right angle to body, elbow straight. Left arm, elbow bent, crosses over body with hand pointing toward right. Left arm is held below right arm.

Take your walk across width of pool where water is chest high. Take each step by crossing the stepping foot over in front of opposite foot, so you move from side to side as well as forward.

As you first step forward with your right foot, swing both arms to opposite side—left arm with straight elbow and right arm with bent elbow; both will point toward left after you have swung them through water.

Continue in this way—each time you place one foot in front of the other, swing both arms to the side opposite the stepping foot.

Variation: For waist and arms. As soon as you have perfected this, try to do it while backing up.

□ **JOGGING, WEIGHT TRAINING, CYCLING, AND RECREATION GROUPS**

Whenever I meet people my age who glow—and their happy number is ever increasing—I usually learn they are runners and super-achievers. Running unravels the knots compounded by demanding work or heavy commitment. And it's such an ego-boosting means of defining your ability to set and carry out a fitness program while maintaining your childhood exuberance. No wonder running is the most addictive exercise of all. A recent magazine blurb declared, "It's better than drugs, better than alcohol, sometimes I swear it's better than sex!"

In my city you cannot park near Balboa Park at lunchtime; too many people have driven up from their offices for their midday run. I walk-jog-run there mornings, Monday through Friday. Weekends, my husband and I spend our fitness hour on the sands of Mission Beach. Just now I'm putting in a jogging path around my own home—an extra pickup for the late evening and for odd hours.

If jogging is new to you, you don't just put on your track shoes and go. Acquire one of the many excellent popular books on the subject. I have a collection of them and subscribe to *Runner's World*. Also I'm a member of the National Jogging Association. It's wise to join a running club, preferably an association-sponsored one. Just about every city has one. Call your Y or athletic club or local university.

All Golden Door guests are given daily instruction in running. Many take the habit home with them. My own program is based on interval training. Begin with a fine stretching warm-up with emphasis on your feet, legs, and thighs. Interval training means you walk so many yards and run so many. You also vary your breathing—deep draughts, short puffs, perhaps breathing through pursed lips. Go through your repertoire of breathing techniques in order to involve all parts of your breathing apparatus.

Never grimace with pain, never suffer one bit. Select your own speed and increase it only as your abilities increase. Begin by walking ten yards and jogging ten. Increase gradually, week by week. At all times you should be able to talk while still running. When I'm jogging along alone I check myself by humming a few bars. To increase your breath capacity, just blow out your breath lustily through your open mouth; then you'll automatically inhale more.

Too, you can vary the run. Mike Spino (*Beyond Jogging, the Inner Spaces of Jogging*) advises you to land on a different part of your foot and to use a different posture. He favors guided fantasy, as well. I have found pleasure in his instruction to imagine a warm hand in the middle of my back and a sky hook holding me tall. What I once felt as tension in my back has become a sense of warm, friendly support.

There are hundreds of physiological reasons, very sound and very sensible, why running is good for your body. Besides, it builds your self-acceptance. And the accompanying euphoria has been likened to Zen, meditation, TM, and mystical experience.

When planning your "where-to's," keep in mind that it is easier to make exercise a habit if the place you have chosen to "work out" is easily accessible.

If weight training is new to you, don't be put off by the notion that you will have to lift one of those big cumbersome weights and, if you are female, that to do so will induce unsightly muscle bulges. Female hormones will protect you from the latter. And big barbells are being supplanted by those neat little ankle and wrist weights. Consider purchasing some if, as you normalize your own weight, you see the necessity for concentrating upon certain contours and muscle groups—particularly upon flabby inner thighs, sagging upper arms, and fatty pads at the shoulders.

Begin by snapping on the smallest size ankle and wrist weights obtainable and then performing your regular exercises, at first very slowly. Later you may wish to experiment with slightly heavier snap-ons.

If you feel the need for a complete body redesign, you may want to consult a recommended gym body conditioner. Just be sure your expert does not require you to work out with motorized equipment. Remember, you should provide the energy to operate the equipment. I am keen on Nautilus and Universal-type gyms; we use the latter at The Golden Door.

Don't neglect cycling. A weekend cycling club is family fun. Some lucky people can cycle to work. Consider keeping your bike at the office. A twenty-minute spin can be a more satisfying tension break than the finest lunch.

This very week discover folk dancing; it's wonderful for "family togetherness." Join a group or start one up with your closest friends. When exercise becomes part of your life-style as sports participation and recreation, it is always the most joyous. Of course, don't neglect ski and hiking clubs. Sierra Club members are always super-fit. Consider your friends, and pick people to share recreational activities rather than cocktail parties.

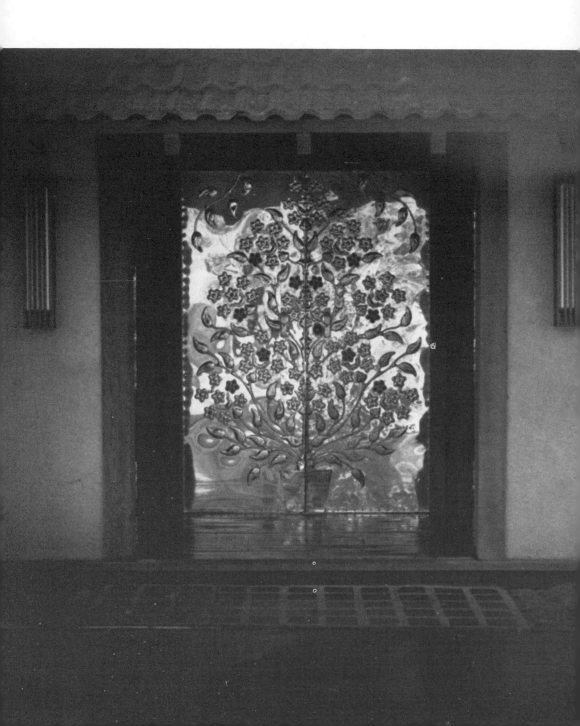

CHAPTER V

NOW, CREATE YOUR OWN GOLDEN DOOR

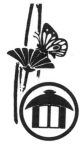
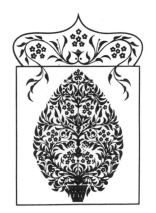
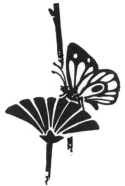

ONE DAY IN THE EARLY 1950s WHEN I WAS WALKING ALONG A path at Rancho La Puerta, I thought I recognized someone who avoided me by ducking behind the gym. "Who was that?" I asked one of the staff. "Oh, that's the lady you were so proud of when she left here four months ago. She is very embarrassed and doesn't want you to see her till she has lost the twenty pounds she regained."

If I were to be proud of my life's work, I saw then, it was vital not to conduct a mere "fat farm" where one takes off a few pounds only to put them on again. I wanted to provide a lasting program that would eliminate from my guests' lives the need to play such a sad game. And so—the philosophy of The Golden Door.

The French phrase—*reculer pour mieux sauter*—comes closest to expressing the essence of The Golden Door: to draw back in order to make a better leap forward. After all that I have said about fitting a program of well-being around your place in the real world, it may seem paradoxical for me now to be advising you to draw back from daily life. But you will have to retreat for a bit so that you may create your own Golden Door.

After her most recent visit, Joan Konner, who has produced so many NBC specials, wrote to thank me for having provided "such a wonderful place for a honeymoon with myself."

"The Golden Door is a heavenly sanctuary," writes Barbara Howar, journalist, television personality, and novelist. She flies out regularly from Washington, D.C.

"I'm so relaxed when I get back," she once confided to *Harper's Bazaar,* "it takes me about six months to start screaming at the children."

Recently she told me, "Everything that happens to me when I leave The Golden Door is wonderful. When I get my stomach flattened and my head straightened, things just seem to come together nicely. All I really need is one more 'pit stop' a year at The Golden Door."

Each of us needs sanctuary. I provide one at The Golden Door by permitting a guest to pause and gather herself in a quiet, remote, otherworldly environment.

The first time Rita Bronowski walked into The Golden Door, it was to escape a devastating emptiness following the sudden death of her husband, Dr. Jacob Bronowski, noted mathematician, scientist, and philosopher whose *Ascent of Man* became a highly praised educational-television series. She sought a refuge where she could deal with her emotions before facing unfamiliar responsibilities.

"I left with a deep sense of The Golden Door's power to heal. It was astonishing that the pressure of all the jobs piling upon me—the unanswered mail, bank details, insurance muddles—seemed lifted."

The second time Rita was a guest at The Golden Door, it was for the purpose of being deliberately "shaken by exercise, jolted completely out of old habits, cleansed mentally and in every sense."

Since then, she has begun to edit several volumes of her late husband's lectures. There's still time daily for a brisk hour-long walk that helps her "feel like a million and ready to tackle it all."

□ I DISCOVERED MY OWN
GOLDEN DOOR

Paradoxical or no, retreating for a serene and solitary weekend has helped me many times to collect my own energies. Since The Golden Door is my business, it can provide no "heavenly sanctuary" for me. Yet there was a time in the late 1950s and early 1960s when I desperately needed a Golden Door-like haven which would give me the time and the perspective to review my life, refill my reservoirs, and make some sense of the future.

I had two very young children and felt tremendously responsible for providing a good life for them, even while I realized I was losing my husband. I knew I would have to be both father and mother.

In addition, I was responsible for running two major health spas. The Golden Door, the second of the two, was just starting on the proverbial shoestring and with all the turmoil attending the birth of any ambitious adventure. My days began at six and ended well past midnight, and every day was a struggle.

I looked at myself and thought, "Well, I can choose to have a nervous breakdown, to get sick, or to do something about it all." I decided to take a long weekend all by myself at a little resort nearby. There was nothing fancy about the place; it was just blessedly quiet.

Just what I was going to do, I didn't know. Because I was too exhausted to take my usual stacks of work, I threw some clothes into a bag along with a Ray Bradbury science-fiction book and—because I had found it lulling reading—Jean-Paul Sartre's *Being and Nothingness.* My state then was not unlike that of three thoroughly vital and very overcommitted women whom I admire, who at one time sought The Golden Door for the same reason—to escape the pressure of excessive demands. When their physicians had prescribed total rest and suggested the hospital, Shana Alexander, Barbara Howar, and Beverly Sassoon came to The Golden Door instead. There, each found within herself her own strengths. Stress studied is the best precondition to change.

At that time, however, I did not realize I was setting up my own

"Lilly tank," my own space for sensory deprivation. I did not know that it also would be my "growth" tank, a refuge where I could think about my life and marshal my strengths.

The first day I did nothing except swim, eat, read science fiction, and gaze into the fire.

The second day I awakened at dawn feeling restless, went for a really long walk, and reached the crest of a small hill just in time for sunrise. So I began my day with a nature high.

After lunching and napping, because I felt good about myself and had nothing else to do, I picked up Sartre and came upon a phrase in *Being and Nothingness* that has given direction to my life: "Freedom is the freedom of choosing but not the freedom of not choosing. *Not to choose is, in fact, to choose not to choose.*"

This simple phrase did it. I knew the choice was mine and that I would elect to lead a different sort of life. By the third day I was driving home, singing happily to myself.

Long ago Socrates said, "The life which is unexamined is not worth living." Pogo more recently said, "We have met the enemy and they is us." I know there are dozens of variations, all leading to the same conclusions. But again I'll quote Sartre, who puts things so well: "A free being is one who makes decisions relating to his past in the light of his future and who does not let himself be determined by the present."

From that day forward, I took responsibility for my life.

Rather than trying to avoid stress, I came to think of it as another term for growth. I saw that I must choose how to react to stress.

◻ *YOUR GOLDEN DOOR*

BEING ALONE CREATIVELY. If, physically, you become what you eat, it follows that, mentally, you become what you think. To encounter yourself, you must do as I did that weekend many years ago. First, get away from your daily life. I suggest that you seek a quiet hotel in the country. Just slip into the hinterland. You shouldn't have to drive more than a hundred miles from home. If your destination has paths to walk along, if there's peace and quiet, you've found your place.

For many people, the prospect of being alone for two days is disconcerting. But only by being alone and allowing the tide of communication to ebb can you see clearly to your own depths and recognize your own patterns. You will treasure the moment when you can be as a solitary pebble dropped in a still pool, and the ripples of thought you release are disturbed by no intrusion.

THE DELIGHTS OF RITUAL.   You've picked out your retreat and set aside the free time. While you are packing, consider two elements that will add to the pleasurable impact of your weekend: ritual and cherishing.

There is a ritual to each aspect of a day at The Golden Door. People are pacing off to classes in their kimonos and warmup suits. All know why they are there, and are in a meditative state beyond thought. There is a sense of serenity and order and purpose.

Cultivate that sense of ritual during your weekend. A simple process like bathing can be turned into a rite. While you are setting out the soap and shampoo and scent and an assortment of different-textured towels, think about the liquid luxury of your bath. Afterward, cherish the bath itself.

Cherish yourself and your reactions to everything that gives you comfort and sustenance.

Start deciding while you pack how many ways you can make the entire weekend a series of rituals. Then you will have freed your energy for other thoughts.

THINGS TO BRING.   You will be doing a lot of walking. Good walking shoes and your favorite old clothes are all you will need. Pack a bathing suit if there is a place to swim.

Also include whatever recreational pleasure-givers are sure to loosen and relax you—but no drugs and no hard liquor. Books are delightful companions. If you are more aural or tactile, bring along a musical instrument, or a sketchpad, or needlepoint, or binoculars for birdwatching—whatever eases you into a peaceful, contemplative state. You must also bring a notebook, a tape measure, and, finally, your calendar for several months past; plus five felt-tipped pens of different colors—black, blue, red, green, and deep lavender. A little later, I'll explain why. You should always keep a personal calendar, and I recommend that you make it as detailed as possible. You need to become aware of the most precious ingredient of life—time.

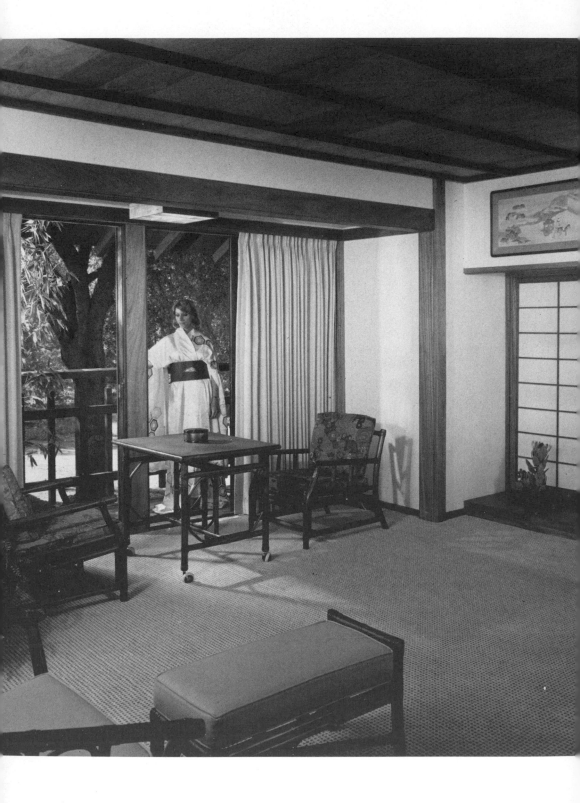

□ *YOUR WEEKEND SCHEDULE*

Friday evening: Arrive, unpack, settle in. Your experience actually begins at dawn on Saturday.

For the time being, revel in the thought that these hours are all your own. Relax. Read, have a glass of wine if you like, and go to sleep early. Set your alarm for sunrise. That is important. You are going to begin afresh, and there is nothing more fresh than a newly created day.

Saturday at dawn: Walk out just as the earliest rays of the sun catch the treetops. Stride out briskly, breathing deeply. Once you feel the warmth of exercise, begin changing the pace. Look around you. Slow down to inspect some special tree or flower, then speed up again until you are breathing strongly and have felt the warm glow that is followed by cooling sweat. Time to slow down again. Alternate for forty minutes; then, back to your room.

8:30 A.M. After cooling off, bathing, and dressing, you probably will be ready for breakfast. Avoid ordering your usual meal. Rather, listen to your body and let it suggest what to eat. Are you really hungry? Early-morning exercise affects people differently. Some come in ravenous, looking for a big farm-style spread. Others have feasted on oxygen and need only a few calories and a little protein to sustain their high. Do whatever feels right but remember that, the bigger the breakfast, the smaller the dinner.

9:00 A.M. For about an hour, find refuge in some sheltered nook. Sit and read, sketch, or play a tune—whatever you enjoy. Experience quietness. Don't think back or ahead. This is a nonthinking day, a turning-off day so that tomorrow can turn you on. We need to leave behind the tyranny of the past, and the dominance of the present, if we are to delight in the future.

10:00 A.M. Now, into movement for about an hour. Your surroundings will suggest the activity: a walk, tennis, horseback riding, swimming, whatever the opportunity affords. Perform vigorously, and at a pace that makes you breathe hard and feel tired but not exhausted.

Alternate being active and quiet throughout the entire weekend; in an analogous way, the weekend itself and others like it will be alternatives to your life's busy-ness and tension. Extend the principle of alternation to almost everything you do. Be conscious of your reactions to bright sunlight as opposed to cool shadows, to input from nature in contrast to occasionally shutting off your perceptions of the physical world. Such contrasts keep us alert and elastic.

11:00 A.M. Time for either a swim or a shower. Don't hurry. Start off with the water mildly warm, then shift to very, very hot, then cool down to icy cold. Feel the water, the cleansing, and the baptismal significance. Dry off slowly and languorously, switching between smooth and rough towels.

11:45 A.M. Devote fifteen minutes to enhancing the body awareness induced by your shower or swim. Wearing as little clothing as you can, find some radio music that suits you. Dance slowly, and later quickly, about the room. Of course you are self-conscious. Acknowledge your feelings, but continue. Stretch out each limb. Be a rag doll and rotate your neck. Shrug your shoulders. Tug on your hair. Massage your scalp muscles. All over your body, tighten and relax each muscle group, one at a time.

12:30 P.M. To lunch. Order something simple, low-calorie, and vegetarian. Have a large fresh-fruit salad with some raisins or nuts, or a vegetable salad and cottage cheese. Eat slowly and consciously, with awareness of the food. Use all your senses. What is the taste, the smell, and the textural feeling of the food in your mouth?

2:00 P.M. You've been up since dawn. You might want a nap after luncheon. Or you might prefer a tour of the area, visits to antique or book stores, or a bicycle ride.

Fine-tune your senses. Let your eye be caught by the curious, the off-beat.

4:00 P.M. You might read or walk. There is no sacred schedule. Just stay with the principle of alternative activities. The morning walk, so many hours ago, set you experiencing the day (not thinking it) in a receptive, sensitive way.

7:00 P.M. Dinner. Indulge yourself. Either order a big meal, with a glass of wine and all the trimmings, to reward yourself for a day well spent; or glow with virtue and tuck into another vegetarian feast.

8:30 P.M. Avoid the desensitizing effect of banal TV programs and the late news. Bring out a book, or light some incense and respond to your favorite music. Don't try to focus very deeply on anything. Then drift off to sleep.

You will have noted, and perhaps with disappointment, that Saturday is a do-nothing, think-nothing day. For the weekend with yourself—to duplicate the special magic of a Golden Door week—you require first the contrast of mindlessness, a time for the pieces to fall apart before you can pick them up and put them together in the way you desire, and thus fashion your life as you wish it to be and to become.

Sunday at dawn: Make this truly the first day of the rest of your life— the day of choices, to be approached with a positive viewpoint. Out you go again for the forty-minute walk that marks the day's beginning. That fresh air, with the high it gives you, is a must for what is to follow.

8:30 A.M. A small breakfast, so you will be alert and sharp.

9:00 A.M. Now you have the whole morning for talking to yourself. Make sure that the you who answers is in a strong and happy mood. If not, skip it. Today is not the day. Negative thoughts and feelings should not be entertained as you set about choosing.

The self-fulfilling prophecy we are planning is the one nature destined you for.

□ *THE IDENTITY INVENTORY*

First, you want the ABC's of yourself. The best way I know to find out what you really think is to write it down. Journalists have a standard formula to ensure that they capture all the essential elements of a story. It consists of five questions, each starting with "W." Ask yourself:

Who are you? Name and address. Married or single. Anything you think is pertinent to a brief physical and psychological description of yourself.

What do you do? This, the first question we put to a stranger, is our way of asking about many other things too. What kind of person are you? What do you believe in? Do you think of yourself as having a job title? What are your patterns of activity? What is your life-style? Your work is the *you* of half your waking day. Your satisfaction with your performance is part of your pride in yourself. Remember that, through work, we handle most of life's anxieties; many of us see our own growth primarily in terms of work.

When is the time factor. It includes your age and your sense of how much future you have. What time is it in your life? Is the dotted line on your life graph curving up or down?

Where are you? Have you a sense of belonging in some one place? Are you rooted or mobile? What paths have you worn across the landscape? Where do you fit in this world?

Why do you do what you do? What is your commitment? Are you in the right place at the right time for you? Do you feel you are doing something valuable, unique? Do you believe in what you are doing? Answer the questions clearly and briefly. Write down your first impulses. They are more likely to be accurate. Study this form as you would a school application or an employment questionnaire. This is your job (life) description. Would you employ yourself? Look inward. What you do today will determine what you will think of yourself as you look back tomorrow.

This is just the first of your own Golden Door Sunday's tasks.

□ *YOUR BODY INVENTORY*

The Body Inventory is equally important, since your mind/body is what puts it all together and makes it all come true.

Ready? Off with your clothes. Begin in front of a mirror. Think of yourself as an artist. Judge the aesthetics of your appearance. Check for harmony, proportion, and vitality. What is the message given by your hair, your eyes, your skin, and your posture? What does the picture tell about the inner you?

Is your mind/body blighted by neglect or radiant with loving concern? Never forget that this is the tool with which you will carve your life.

Chart your own country. Write down your weight and your height. Measure your hips, waist, and bust or chest. Use these body statistics as a starting point rather than as a means of comparing yourself to Perfect Person.

Form an idea of how much excess fat/fuel you're carrying; visualize those extra pounds. Take them off with your mind's eye and set them down, *there,* on the table. Heavy, aren't they? Of course they have been slowing you down, both physically and emotionally. Each pound represents more unnecessary work for your heart and lungs. If you are average, you will live into your late seventies. What will your life, physically, be like then? This too is a decision you're making today.

Although appearance tells a lot, even more revealing is your body's response to activity. So you must measure your body's endurance, flexibility, and strength.

ENDURANCE (THE STEP TEST).   Good health is more than skin deep. The endurance that gives you steady, glowing vitality under stress comes from your cardiovascular/respiratory system.

Sit down and relax for a minute or two, then take your pulse (count for thirty seconds and multiply by two). Do it again to check the accuracy of your count. This is your resting heart rate. Write it down.

Next comes a test of your heart's response to physical exertion. The President's Council on Physical Fitness recommends the two-minute Step Test for this purpose. It is not difficult. It informs you how quickly your heart returns to normal after exertion, and is a simple test of circulatory efficiency.

You perform the Step Test by stepping up and down, onto a bench, chair, or step fifteen to seventeen inches high. Here is how the President's Council bulletin describes the Step Test:

> Count One—Place right foot on bench.
> Count Two—Bring left foot alongside right, and stand erect.
> Count Three—Lower right foot to floor.
> Count Four—Lower left foot to floor.
> Repeat the four-count movement thirty times a minute for two minutes, then take your pulse. Write it down. Now rest for two minutes, and again take your pulse. (You can find the pulse by applying middle and index fingers of one hand firmly to the inside wrist of the other hand, on the thumb side.) Record the count.
> Rest again for two minutes and take your pulse, recording it for future comparisons.

As your lifelong fitness program progresses, you will find your heart becomes more efficient. The measure of that efficiency will be a lower pulse rate on the first measurement after stepping, and less of a difference between that and the second measurement. As the difference between the two decreases, you see the approach of fitness. (Take future tests at about the same time of day, and use a bench or chair of the same height.)

Endurance develops slowly. You can, however, make yourself appreciably more flexible in just a few days.

FLEXIBILITY. Stand straight, feet twelve inches apart, arms hanging loosely. Bend forward slowly, knees straight, and try to touch your toes. Do not lunge or strain; stop when you feel pain. Do it again with a tape measure. Write down the distance from your extended fingertips to your toes. If you can't touch your toes now, you should be able to within a very few weeks after starting your stretching and limbering exercises (see Body Awakeners, pages 104–140). Eventually you may be able to touch your toes without flexing your knees. But don't push for this if you are stiff or have a history of back trouble. Very easy does it.

Now test your hips. Hold one arm out in front of you with the palm of your hand about six inches above waist height. Now swing up the leg on that same side, and try to touch your big toe to the hand, keeping your knee straight. You should be able to swing your leg forward above the horizontal. If you're stiff, it's most likely because you haven't been using certain joints, tendons, and ligaments, and partly because of tension in the body. It is a condition that improves quickly as you work on it.

STRENGTH. Strength in the abdominal area is important, since those muscles directly affect posture. The simplest test for abdominal strength is the sit-up. Lie on your back with your knees comfortably bent and your arms above your head. Sit up. Count the number of times you can do it. Write them down.

Now test your arm power with knee push-ups. Lie on your stomach, hands under your shoulders. Keeping your back straight, use your arms to push yourself up until, with arms extended, your weight rests on your hands and knees. How many can you do? Write down the total.

Finally, the leg muscles. Stand on your toes, back against the wall, arms horizontal in front of you. With your back straight, bend your knees and *squat* with your buttocks no lower than your knees. Then come back up to a standing position. How many times can you do this? Write down the total.

You now have a sheet of figures for weight, height, hips, waist, and bust; for heart rate at rest, immediately after a Step Test, two minutes after, and four minutes after; for toe touches; for sit-ups, knee push-ups, and squats—and you now have a much more finely tuned sense of your own body than you had an hour ago.

WATCH YOURSELF GROW YOUNGER. Now make a note on your calendar to take another Body Inventory at the end of next month. After that, inventory every three months. As you compare each set of new figures with the old ones, you can watch yourself grow younger. As you begin to watch your results and feel the impact of fitness on your daily life you will be surprised at your behavior modification. Just like Skinner's pigeons, you will be enticed by immediate gratification. You will start—again I quote from Sartre—"to obey nature in order to command it."

Almost lunch time. Stretch out your body. Go for a walk, swim, or any form of exercise that offers a change. Then to lunch.

□ *LIFE'S COLORS ON YOUR CALENDAR*

Of all the tricks of the trade I've found useful in forty years in the health business, the one my guests most appreciate is this simple use of the calendar. I suggest that each guest thus commemorate, each month, the day she arrived home from The Golden Door, because it is the start of a new life. I hope you too will want to commemorate the day you read the last page, close this book, and continue on your chosen path.

In the early afternoon, study your calendar as you might study your face. It's you—your time, your day. How you use all this determines your life. Look at the map of your life as it was. Now decide what to keep, what to discard, and what to change.

"Those who cannot remember the past are condemned to repeat it," said George Santayana. To plan your future, you must analyze your past. You must avoid the pitfalls of wishful thinking, the over-idealistic resolutions which we all hope for and rarely achieve, if you are to be realistic and *successful*. Consider the recent month you believe to be most typical. You are going to use this month to keep from floating off into rationalizations. Now underline each calendar entry as follows:

Black for everything you did that you didn't like, that was a waste of your time: a board or committee that you're not contributing anything to, a shopping trip that could have been handled by telephone, an assignment that someone else at work could have carried out, a luncheon that was a bore.

Blue for duty: earning money, chores, family responsibilities, and the like. Certain things are necessities. The more you dislike doing them, the faster you should get them done.

Red for what you contributed to your health and physical well-being: a brisk walk, tennis, even a trip to the beauty shop.

Green for growth, your personal growth, every new dimension that has added to the width and breadth of your life. Plant any seed, it will sprout, germinate, grow. Remove the growth elements, it will die. So do we, each in our own way.

Lavender for everything that was joyous. In my childhood, it seemed to me that healthy meant happy. There was so much laughter and song around the evening bonfires of the New York Hiking Club, and, later, on the black sandy beaches of Tahiti.

Today, I seldom hear enough laughter, except among children or my rejuvenated guests, working out all those tensions on the exercise mats at The Golden Door.

Joy, like the bluebird of Maeterlinck, needs to be sought out. Joy can best be found at home but you have to create the right environment if joy is to thrive. For your health and growth and joy, every day should be rainbow-hued. Study your patterns. See where you can convert some of your blacks and some of your blues into reds, greens, and lavenders.

Be creative about it. Bicycling instead of driving will change some chores from black to red. Lunch in the park with a friend, instead of a hurried-up sandwich at your desk, turns out lavender. Of course, many blues are going to remain as they are. But you can intersperse them with reds and greens. They all serve to balance your day, providing more contrast and more pleasure to each alternating period.

Apply this principle to household duties, to office, and other tasks. Just as there needs to be an ecological balance in nature, so too there must be a balance in Man.

Do not be tempted to add up the blacks, the blues, and the reds. But once again, a month from this day, reserve a quiet time for your calendar and yourself. Take out your colored pens and repeat the process. Again, do not add, do not judge your performance, but do review your Life Calendar month after month. The day will come when you will mentally color each entry as you write, and you will then realize you are the author of your own life's history and can make it read as you wish.

Because I'm thriving in all my worlds, my growth weekends now serve me differently. Yet, as each new decade of my life comes along, I take such a weekend again and again. As I've said, I was a June bride when I was fifty—a decision that required several weekends. That, too, was the year my youngest child became a freshman in high school. Every mother must spend some time deliberating how she plans to function once the nest is empty.

Today we are living longer than ever in history. The average man and woman have a third more time to walk this earth and leave their imprint. More and more people realize that twenty to twenty-five years is enough at one job, and mid-life career changes will soon become the rule. We will look forward to scholarships and not pensions. It behooves us to stretch out our middle years with a good fitness program so that we may remain productive and physically capable of grasping new options.

□ *L'ENVOI*

Your visit to your own Golden Door is about to end. Do a bit more thinking. Give yourself a real chance for success. If you draw up some lovely goals that are impossible to attain, you will wind up frustrated and no happier than before. Be realistic. Your goals must not only be possible and plausible, but specific, and set month by month. If you have asked too much of yourself, don't feel guilty. Begin as slowly as you must.

Review the habit patterns on which you have built your life to date. Save a few, and work to discard others so that you can fill your days with new being. You will sleepwalk through life if you repeat your days until there are none.

Use the present to prophesy your future. You must choose your life, just as you choose the thoughts you welcome and later reflect upon.

Remember, as Thomas Dulguff of the Menninger Foundation says, "It's easier to act your way into a new way of thinking, than to think your way into a new way of acting."

You, and my guests, very well might ask, "But is this much work really necessary?" That is the decision you alone can make. What kind of life do you need if you are to find happiness? What is your image of yourself today? What would you like it to be tomorrow? What kind of relationship with yourself do you wish to achieve?

As you perceive yourself, so you will become.

CHAPTER VI

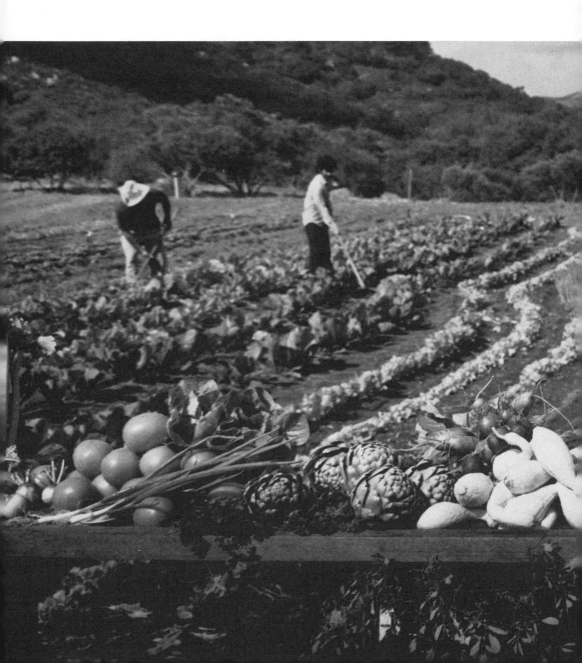

GLORIOUS EATING: THE GOLDEN DOOR WAY TO MAKE FOOD YOUR FRIEND

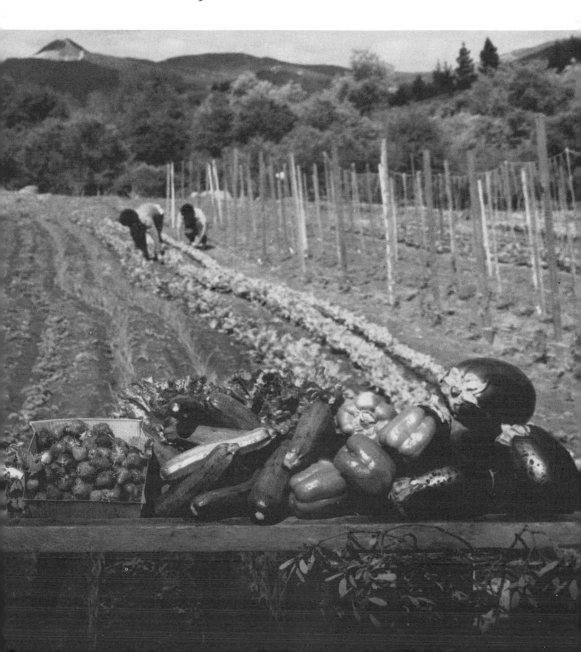

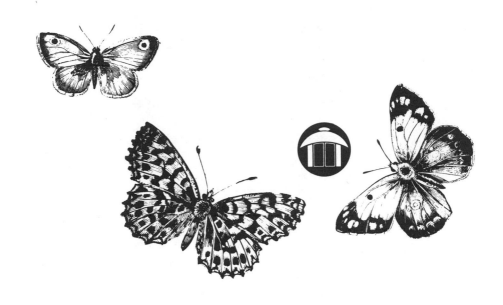

ANYONE WHO HAS EVER LINGERED BESIDE A NEWSSTAND KNOWS how preoccupied Americans are with food and diet. One cannot help being aware of it—and confused as well. Whom to believe?

Do not worry. My work requires that I make the time to keep up with the latest opinions of all the experts. As I pass on to you their consensus I also will be advising you how to pleasure yourself as you grow in your ability to balance your intake of proper food/fuel with your output of living energy. Learning to live with the right food is not at all a grim matter. If you learn my lessons well you'll have learned to discard your attitude of crime and punishment, or gorge and diet.

173

□ A GAME PLAN FOR LIFE

Appetite is nature's way of ensuring survival; loving food is part of loving life. Since eating is something you must do daily in order to sustain life, be demanding of the food you eat. It should taste very good and be very, very good for you. You must arrange a better way of eating that's both normal for you and consistent with your physical size and activity age and with the weight you think ideal.

My joy was immense when I read in early 1977 a report by the Senate Select Committee on Nutrition and Human Needs.* It said exactly what we've been preaching during the past several decades.

In effect, the report stated that Americans should go back to the old days and eat fruits, vegetables, and grains instead of relying on fats and sugars for 60 percent of their food energy. Our eating habits may be "as profoundly damaging to the nation's health as the widespread contagious diseases of the early part of the century." Rapidly increasing fat consumption has "been linked to six of the ten leading causes of death. . . . Too much fat, too much sugar or salt can be and are linked directly to heart disease, cancer, obesity and stroke, among other killer diseases."

A 40 percent drop in sugar consumption, a 12 percent reduction in fat consumption, and a restriction of salt intake could reduce heart disease by 25 percent, cancer by 20 percent, and infant mortality by 50 percent.

In addition to substituting increased consumption of fruits, vegetables, and grains for high-level sugar and fat consumption, Americans should eat less meat and more poultry and fish, drink nonfat milk rather than whole milk, and consume fewer high-cholesterol foods. In fact, cholesterol consumption should drop by half, to about 300 milligrams daily.

Such a diet would not only supply vitamins and micronutrients inexpensively, but could also reduce the risk of heart disease, and lower the incidence of bowel cancer by producing more fiber.

* By all means send at once for the report, "Dietary Goals for the United States." Write to The Superintendent of Documents, U.S. Government Printing Office, Washington, D.C. 20402. Enclose 95¢. Stock No. 052-070-03913-2.

The committee report is the first comprehensive statement by any branch of the federal government on the risks involved in the American diet, and most unexpected in a government document are the following two statements.

From Mary Goodwin, public health nutritionist:

> The pleasures of seeing, smelling and tasting food that looks, smells and tastes good, nourish the personality with sensuous experience even as the vitamins and minerals are making their contribution to the growth of bone and muscle. An awareness of real people preparing and serving the foods helps too.
>
> Which is to say that if you eat enough precooked, frozen, reheated foil-and-plastic packed lunches out of machines, part of you will starve to death.

And from Dr. Bruno Bettelheim, noted child psychiatrist:

> Eating and being fed are intimately connected with our deepest feelings. They are the basic interactions between human beings on which rest all later evaluations of oneself, of the world, and of our relationship to it. Eating experiences condition our entire attitude to the world, not so much because of how nutritious is the food we are given, but because of the feelings and attitudes with which it is given.

☐ FAD AND FACT AND FANCIES

You've noticed that this chapter head uses the word "food"—not "diet." And you've already gathered why. I simply don't believe in denial, which diets entail.

Hear about crash diets from Cristina Delorean, one of the world's most beautiful and highly paid photographic models. "They make me sick," she says.

Her face was on the cover of eight national magazines last year and is seen repeatedly in current advertisements for a leading cosmetics company. With all that going for her, she was still battling our country's most pervasive beauty problem—overweight.

"I weighed too much for fashion modeling," she explains. "My face was okay, but I couldn't do clothes."

The nagging conviction that she was overweight frustrated her into a series of crash diets, all of them bad. "After a few days on one of those diets, I would begin to get dizzy and then start vomiting," she remembers. "I had to do something sensible."

One day she read an issue of *Town and Country* magazine devoted entirely to health and beauty spas. (Her picture was on the cover.) After studying the articles, she made a reservation at The Golden Door.

> I went expecting two weeks of aggravating diet and exercise. Within about four or five days I began to feel better than I had in a long, long time. By the second week, I felt better than I ever had in my whole life. I was a new person. It was a revelation that a well-balanced, low-calorie diet could taste good and be good for you.

When she left, Cristina took home Golden Door assets to share with her family. Her husband, John Delorean, is an automobile designer and manufacturer. They have a four-year-old son, Zachary. Cristina notes:

> Modeling is hard work. It demands a lot of muscle control, and I have to be on my feet a good part of the day. I use Golden Door exercises to ease the pressure. No matter how tired I am when I come home from work, I get down on the floor and exercise. It gets my blood going and gives me my second wind. I feel great.

I'd no more urge a crash diet upon you than I would upon Cristina. What you must arrange is a better way of eating—one that's normal for you, as you are now, with your already established life-style.

The so-called "newer" and "better" diets inevitably prove to be just a better way of deviling yourself with some new denial. Each new fad diet—like the others—is a game of Russian roulette. It may not kill you, but it produces new tensions and unhappiness by dictating that you sit in on a punishment game instead of a reward game.

I know whereof I speak because for many years I tried every new diet plan on my guests. Fortunately, one at last runs out of mistakes. What we have discovered with our guests at The Golden Door is an affirmative, creative way to *intensify* the pleasure you derive from sane quantities of really delectable food. The goal, after all, is not cessation of eating.

There is a folk tale—Romanian or Hungarian, depending upon who tells it—that says everything that needs to be said:

> A traveler was walking down a road when he saw a peasant leaning against a tree and weeping as if his heart had broken.
> "What is wrong?" the traveler asked. "Why are you weeping?"
> "My perfect horse!" the peasant sobbed. "It died!"
> "Ah. What made your perfect horse perfect?"
> For a while the peasant was too overcome to speak. Then at last he raised his head. "I worked with that horse for months. Oh, he cooperated so willingly! Every day he would eat a little less of my oats, less and less, until finally he got to the point where he became the perfect farm animal. He didn't have to eat at all. Nothing. Not a handful of oats, not a blade of grass.
> "And then—a catastrophe! An unimaginable misfortune! Just as he became perfect, he died."

□ *FIGURING THE TOTAL CALORIES*

The pleasure you experience from appropriate food can transform your looks, your health, and the overall stimulus that life brings you.
Food satisfies three basic needs:

1. Energy, to propel you
2. Delight, to motivate you
3. Nutrition, to build and maintain your body

Are your present eating habits truly fulfilling all these needs? Being active and exuberant, mixing out there in the world with all your ebullience and vitality is going to be vastly more worthwhile for you than anxiously counting calories. Never be intimidated by the word *calorie* and what it represents. It's only a specific measure of energy, after all . . . the amount of heat necessary to raise one gram of water one degree centigrade.

If you count only the physical calories in your diet you may always believe yourself hungry. But food also provides psychological calories. The magnificent San Diego Zoo utilizes diet pellets containing all the nutrients that each species of animal is known to need. Yet I was fascinated to see a special note at the bottom of the prescribed diet. It was labeled "For Delight," and listed apples, bananas, and certain fresh leaves. When I asked a zoo veterinarian what would happen if the animal didn't receive this special supplement, he said, "The coat becomes dull. Stools are irregular. Either there are almost no offspring or the offspring are deformed. The animal develops muscular problems. And, worst of all—he bites his keeper."

When you combine the physical calorie with the psychological calorie, you have what I call the Total Calorie, which I picture as a sort of iceberg. The visible top 10 percent is the physical calorie. It's supported by the invisible 90 percent, the psychological calorie.

If the calorie's impact were purely physical, Metrecal would be bigger than I.T.T., and everyone would be content to select from the 50 basic foods once offered at the country general store, rather than from the 15,000 seductive variations now cunningly set out on your supermarket's shelves to entice you. (Supermarkets understand enough about the psychological calorie to capitalize on it for their own purposes. Be wary. Consider the breakfast cereal, cute packaging aside. Today's 180 cereals still are made from just 8 basic grains.)

Since eating is an act of intake, you are open and vulnerable not only to food but to suggestion. Hence the business or social lunch where, with your defenses down, you can easily be talked into something you would rather not do.

Food takes care of emotional needs that are real and profound. By all means make food your friend—but by no means your *only* friend. Really serious weight problems usually belong to the men and women who forsake all other gratifications for those of the table.

□ *LESS IS MORE*

Over the years at The Golden Door we have perfected a variety of techniques for making a relatively small amount of food immensely satisfying. You can enhance your enjoyment by following them.

1. *Less is more* if you continue to eat whatever you genuinely like. If you really detest something—even though somebody has told you it's a wonder food—don't eat it. Especially in times of stress, it's important that you retain familiar flavors, textures, and cooking fragrances at mealtime.

Hold onto all your pet recipes, but serve the "main course" on the salad plate and the salad on the dinner plate. If steak is a dinner favorite, the accompaniment should be something lean like zucchini. Reserve baked potatoes for fish or soufflé nights. If spaghetti is the side dish, it's time for clear soup, green salad, and a dessert of fruit. When there's a birthday cake, all the other courses should be low in calories. This way you can eat what you've always been fond of and yet not add unwanted pounds. It's all merely a matter of balancing total intake.

2. *Less is more* when you consciously eat in very agreeable surroundings and without distractions. Infrequently, I hear a Golden Door guest complain of hunger. I always check to see if she has eaten in her room. Almost invariably, she has. Gulping down almost-unnoticed food while reading or sitting in bed is no way to savor it.

At home, standing by the refrigerator and eating is one of the best means of getting fat without really enjoying the food. And newspapers and television are dreadful mealtime partners, literally specters at the feast. All these distractions mean that you'll entertain only a momentary sort of gullet pleasure which doesn't last long; soon you're hungry again.

Even if you're eating alone, favor yourself with the sensuous delights of flowers, a cheerful tray, and your best china. Carry your food out of the kitchen and into a harmonious setting. Augment it with music.

3. *Less is more* when you eat with agreeable people, whether family or friends. Conversation and companionship make food seem even more satisfying. Always take care at table to keep all conversation upbeat and interesting. Avoid feuding at all costs. Dinnertime, usually, is the only hour of the day when the entire family can sit down to share a happy experience. Make it happy for everyone, including yourself.

4. *Less is more* when you open your senses in new directions. Normal as it is to find gratification in food, it is dangerous to depend on it for most of your rewards. You must seek out others. Make a point of scheduling daily pleasures for yourself—a new hairdo, a scarf, a record, a get-away-from-it-all swim—things you can arrange casually, without effort. Instead of dreaming of exquisite menus and Brillat-Savarin fêtes, settle for a frequent bubble bath, a new book, a concert, or a movie. Assume a gourmet attitude toward *all* of living, and you'll have little trouble adhering to your new diet plan.

And consider this: When you're uncomfortable or bored, your body

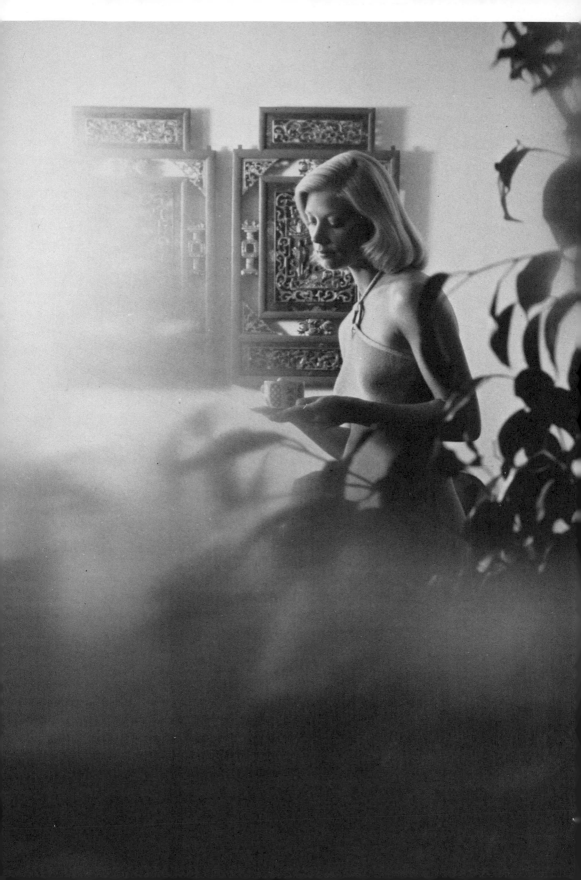

relays signals of dissatisfaction which are often mistaken for hunger. Actually, you then may need a change of pace—a splash of cold water on your face or a quick brisk walk.

As for true hunger, it can come to be your friend if you learn to associate the sensation with good looks and vitality and with pride in your body.

□ *BEGINNING YOUR FOOD PLAN*

Before you can improve your eating patterns you must be thoroughly aware of them.

1. TAKE A CLOSE LOOK AT HOW YOU EAT. For three days write down everything, how much, when, where, with whom. Do you nibble and snack, or eat one big meal; if you snack, is it from the time you begin to prepare dinner until bedtime? Do you dine out often? Do you eat with the family, or from a solitary tray? In the kitchen, bedroom, dining room, living room? While you read or watch TV? In the beginning count every physical calorie so you'll have an accurate picture of your intake—per meal and per day. (At any bookstore and many newsstands you can buy one of those inexpensive paperbacks listing the calories contained in standard servings of almost every imaginable food. My favorite is *Calories and Carbohydrates* by Barbara Kraus.)

2. SELECT YOUR ACTIVITY AGE. Look closely at both sides of the energy equation: Calorie *intake* (ideally) equals energy *output*. Laborers, for example, and many teen-agers and professional athletes who burn up terrific amounts of energy in their daily activities can consume five or six thousand calories a day—two or three times as much as the average thirty-five-year-old American would dare—without gaining weight.

If you eat as much as you always have and don't step up your exercise, you'll add fat. If you heedlessly allow yourself to grow older with your intake at the same level, the gradual changes in your output eventually will unbalance your system. So think. Even if you're younger now, by allowing yourself to gain a pound a year at each Christmas dinner you'll be twenty pounds overweight when you blow out the forty candles on your cake.

To be more specific: if you consume an excess of only ninety-six calories a day (the equivalent of one slice of bread), in five years you could conceivably be fifty pounds overweight. In contrast, the weight gain could have been prevented if only twenty-five minutes of brisk walking had been added to each day. And don't forget that the benefits of exercise continue long after you have stopped moving. So *do* walk a few extra blocks and up the stairs before sitting in that office chair, both in the morning and again at lunch. Walking a brisk mile each day for thirty-five days is a simple way to lose a pound—walk more and you will lose more. Those who are overweight have an even greater potential for losing weight since it takes more energy to move two hundred pounds than one hundred pounds.

Your body is not a statistic. That's why I'm not including a "Recommended Calories Per Day by Weight and Age" chart, nor a "Recommended Weight by Height and Age." I don't believe in them. The mirror is your surest measuring stick, and the bathroom scale is your best daily gauge.

3. RELATE YOUR INTAKE TO YOUR BODY SIZE. The logic of this is impressed upon us very early when someone first reads us the story of "Goldilocks and the Three Bears" . . .

In a neat little cottage in the midst of a deep woods there once lived three bears. One was a great big daddy bear, one was a middle-sized mama bear, and one was a wee little baby bear.

One morning Mother Bear made a big batch of porridge for breakfast. She filled a great big bowl for daddy bear, a middle-sized bowl for her middle-sized self, and a wee little bowl for baby bear.

I'm appalled at the civilized nonsense called "portion control," a measured serving for the mythical average man. This evil is practiced in every school, restaurant, and hospital in the country, and in most homes. A flagrant illustration of this was told me by Stephen McClintock, the physiologist who administered my stress test to me:

"I'm six feet, six inches tall, and in the Army where you line up to be served, I followed a four-foot-six soldier. No matter how I pleaded for food, I was told, 'Everyone is treated equally in the Army.' So I got skinnier and skinnier and my messmate got fatter and fatter."

Vivid Bess Myerson, thirty years ago the nation's stunning beauty queen, and now our leading advocate for consumer protection, has developed a personal approach. "Snacks are the enemy," she says, knowing exactly where she stands in this controversy.

Bess is a busy woman, and her remarkable career continues to embrace the widest range of roles: TV and radio commentator; newspaper and magazine writer/editor; lecturer, teacher, and consultant to consumer and industry associations. As Commissioner of Consumer Affairs for New York City, she pioneered many consumer-protection programs which have been adopted by numerous cities.

She makes the point that people as busy and on-the-go as most of us today have two basic problems—to find the time to eat, and to find the willpower to eat correctly. "It isn't easy in our snack society," she says:

> "Grabbing a bite to eat" may do wonders for our daily timetables but it certainly doesn't do much for our health—or our hips. That kind of tension—which is a sign of our times—can unbalance a diet. The Golden Door helped me get the balance back. Its good food and good sense about food can strengthen even the most lagging of willpowers. It isn't enough for any of us to know about food and nutrition and additives, and the value of exercise, and the rules of health that we break at our own peril. We also have to know the places and opportunities which make it easier for us to do more than just think about those things, while we are running around and snacking ourselves into trouble.
>
> I looked for those places and opportunities—and I found one. Behind The Golden Door, you might say. My willpower is doing nicely, thank you.

4. MAKE YOUR OWN FOOD PLAN. Tailor a program to suit yourself; go on making alterations and adjustments till it fits you exactly.

My lawyer friend John Rhoades developed his own individualistic slant on dieting:

"From Monday to Friday I eat sparingly: a light breakfast, not too much lunch, and very little dinner. I promise myself that from Friday night until Sunday night I can eat anything I want. All week I look forward to the bonus weekend when I can drink my beer and eat Mexican food and lasagna and all that." Certainly not a utopian diet plan, but if it works for him, that's all that counts. Let me add that John, who lives by the sea, runs three miles every morning on the beach and takes a quick swim before work. He weighs less today than when he joined the Navy years ago.

5. DON'T BE IMPATIENT. Don't be too ambitious. Your eating habits took years to form. Long-established habits can't be altered overnight, nor should they be.

6. SELECT A MANAGEABLE GOAL. You remember my tricks of a ten percenter: eat 10 percent less, exercise 10 percent more, and think 10 percent more. It's a very low-pressure game that nevertheless will bring you out on top at year's end, like a sound conservative investment. The thinking calls for you to outwit yourself in little ways. Examples: make 4 ounces of morning orange juice into 8 ounces by diluting it with 50 percent water; use really small dishes—they can be a great help in making less seem like more. Begin your meal with a bulky low-calorie salad or a clear soup.

The result, as I have figured out, is that if you eat 10 percent fewer calories all year, you can have a few weekend bacchanalia and still weigh less than you would otherwise.

7. REMEMBER THE PSYCHOLOGICAL CALORIE, particularly at the end of the day. When we discuss their "take-out" plan before guests leave The Golden Door, I always question them closely about dinner habits and usually make major changes there.

People—and in particular people who work—frequently do very well all during the day and then blow it with the nonstop dinner. Those who cook often sit down to their second dinner because they've already eaten the first while nibbling by the stove.

When you come home starved and you still have dinner to prepare, recognize that your food plan is in peril and grab an immediate blood-sugar raiser—a real tension-breaker: a cup of tea, with a few sunflower seeds and raisins; a sliced pear or apple spread with peanut butter; two or three tiny crackers with cheese and a cup of hot bouillon. Jump into a very, very hot shower, followed by a cold one to wash away the tensions of the day. Take a very quick and vigorous walk, even if you can spare only ten minutes, before returning to the kitchen and your dinner preparations. Feel the tension dissolve.

□ THE CALORIE GAME:
FIGURING THE PERCENTAGES

Once you have probed your eating habits (and certain other personal tendencies), we'll assume you've decided to reduce your intake of physical calories.

A good rule of thumb when combining food and exercise facts is to remember the estimate that a pound of fat is worth 3,500 calories. In figuring out your own weight-loss schedule, you may assume that for every 3,500 calories you either don't swallow, or burn away, you can eliminate one pound of real fat—not just a pound of water that will return the next day.

By trimming off just 100 of your daily calories, you can lose that full pound of fat in 35 days. Slow, but you do need nutrients and the satisfactions of the Total Calorie. If you cut back too far, you may feel malnourished, uneasy, and unhappy. That's why at The Golden Door, where the most controlled circumstances prevail, the weight-loss diet is rarely permitted to drop below a daily average of 800 calories. (See menus, pages 211–281.) If you're at home and taxed by the usual mundane stresses and you're a middle-sized, middle-aged female, you shouldn't let your daily total slip below 1,250 calories. For a middle-sized, middle-aged male, 1,800 calories is the desirable minimum. Let exercise do its share in the weight-loss program. It is a fact that it is easier for a man to lose weight on more food than it is for a woman. Because of his size, a man requires more calories just to maintain minimal body functions. Women have a higher proportion of fat cells, and consequently a lower proportion of cell-mass (muscle mass) than men; and as we age, watch out!—for the total cell-mass continues to *decrease* as the years *increase*.

The energy requirements of the body depend on the basal metabolic rate which is affected by both the degree of physical activity and the body size. The basal metabolic rate is the measurement of energy output when one is in a state of complete rest, and it depends on the total cell-mass. To simplify it all, think of the cell-mass as that which consumes energy, speeding you up, and fat cells as those which store energy, slowing you down.

A proper balance of vigorous exercise and both the correct amounts and quality of food is a must. Whatever your age, you need to begin now.

At The Golden Door we apportion our calories differently from just about every other authority on food. That's because we want you to save your precious calories and to schedule Lucullan rewards for the hour of the day when you need them most. We want you to ensure yourself the most gratification, the most relaxation, the most opportunity for communicating meaningfully with someone else as you dine. In other words, we advise you to hold out for hedonism of a mild sort.

CALORIE APPORTIONMENT

For those who prefer their weight loss short and snappy:

- ☐ Breakfast .... 10 percent
- ☐ Luncheon .... 20 percent
- ☐ Dinner .... 70 percent

For those who are patient and willing to persevere:

- ☐ Breakfast .... 20 percent
- ☐ Luncheon .... 30 percent
- ☐ Dinner .... 50 percent

☐ *BREAKFAST*

Allotting 10 or 20 percent for breakfast may not seem like much, but these days who has time for more? If you're allowing yourself 1,250 calories for the full day, this will amount to either 125 or 250 for the morning meal—just enough to lift the blood sugar and start you off. (If you're exercising on the morning pattern, as explained in the Movement chapter (page 32), thirty minutes of satisfying exercise movement may assuage hunger. You've already feasted on oxygen!)

I've been told most people do better on a more substantial breakfast, and there's no reason for you to be married forever to a skimpy one. But The Golden Door's very successful weight-loss plan always has been predicated on just a few morning calories. You've rested all night, you have unwound, and you don't need a lot of stoking in the morning. The whole day is ahead—a marvelous blank check on which you can fill in anything you want.

Yes, I've read the late, influential Adelle Davis's recommendation of big breakfasts. She argued so persuasively that for a week I drew up elaborate breakfast menus—but to no one's benefit, for in my house, and quite possibly in yours, there's no one around on weekday mornings to relish a sizable meal. How many people are disposed to linger and chat in the mornings?

You can turn out a tasty 150-calorie starter with half a cantaloupe and ½ ounce of Monterey Jack cheese on half a slice of homemade wheat toast; or a grated apple with cinnamon, raisins, bran, and a few chopped nuts; or ½ cup of yogurt with wheat germ and a few raisins; or a cracker spread with cottage cheese and cinnamon, slipped under the broiler; or some invention of your own. Sip your tea without sugar. If coffee is your drink, you'll want to replace it with a decaffeinated version because you'll not be needing stimulants.

People often approach me to ask, "What is the right diet for me?" as if I carried diet regimens like color swatches to be quickly matched to the proper person.

The only satisfactory answer to this question is a complex answer. In her book, *Between Heaven and Earth,* my friend Laura Huxley suggests that you cannot determine the right diet for yourself until you first have answered questions such as these:

Where do you live? How old are you? What kind of job do you have?

Is your sex life satisfactory? How do you feel toward yourself? With whom do you eat? What is your last thought at night? Are you in love? What is your first thought in the morning?

Do you have children? Is the intensity of your emotional feeling markedly different before and after a meal? Is your sense of smell a keen guide, or do you hardly notice it? Do you breathe consciously sometimes?

Do you meditate? Do you have a totally satisfactory relationship with one or more persons? Are you now living in a condition physically, psychologically, or emotionally stressful?

Laura concludes: "Your answers to these and other questions, coordinated with your genetic heritage and chemical analysis, are basic to your choice of diet and of food supplements." *

In any event, your breakfast should include some form of substantial whole grain, for the B-complex vitamins and the indispensable trace minerals. The whole grains should be as close to their natural state as possible (remember, bread once was called the Staff of Life).

The Golden Door food plan leans heavily on raw fresh fruits and vegetables and natural whole grains. All of these contain as many extraordinary unknown life-giving substances as they do known ones.

I agree with the current emphasis on fibrous foods. They always have been a precondition to an easy process of peristalsis (contractions by which the intestines force their contents onward). Furthermore, fibrous foods are acclaimed for their ability to hold moisture, the natural lubricant of the intestinal tract, whereas overprocessed foods induce constipation.

At Rancho La Puerta as well as The Golden Door, it cannot be said that the serving of fibrous foods is enjoying a revival. At neither place did they ever go into a decline.

□ *LUNCHEON*

THE APPETITE SPOILER.   Remember your mother telling you, "Don't eat anything before dinner; it will spoil your appetite!"? Well, Mom was right. And we recommend systematic appetite spoilers before each noon and evening meal. The appetite spoiler will begin to raise the blood-sugar level, sending impulses to inform the brain that the body has been fed. This process requires a full thirty to forty minutes. During a low-calorie meal it's desirable to recognize that the process is taking place. Then you can silently monitor your rising blood-sugar level and know that soon you won't feel a bit hungry. The spoiler can contribute a head start and shorten the gnawing gap between mealtime and its resultant satisfaction.

LUNCHEON STRETCHERS.   Here again, 250 or 375 calories for lunch isn't generous, but you can make it seem so.

* *Between Heaven and Earth.* Laura Archera Huxley. New York: Farrar, Straus, and Giroux, 1975.

It's imperative to take luncheon in two courses. At home, lead off with an appetizer—your appetite spoiler. It can be a serving of berries, or celery stuffed with pot cheese, or a bowl of consommé, or a tomato-and-onion salad served with almost no dressing—just something low-calorie to set off the physiological process. Wait fifteen minutes. Make some phone calls. Open your junk mail. Inspect your garden.

If you work in an office, have your spoiler just as you leave to take your lunch hour. Nibble sunflower seeds and a small apple, or eat a half-cup of plain yogurt. Then walk to the restaurant. If you have spent 75 calories on the appetite spoiler, you still have 175 to 300 calories for the rest of your luncheon.

And now the luncheon, itself.

Each noon, crisp up your energy with a different and large mixed vegetable salad. Top it with one of our dressings, or one of your own. That might be oil and wine vinegar, or lemon juice, with seasonings and a grated, hard-cooked egg; yogurt with curry powder, salt, and pepper; yogurt with crumbled blue cheese, plus seasonings. When vegetables are truly fresh, little more is necessary. I love to add a bit of French mustard or horseradish, and great salad herbs are fresh or dried mint, tarragon, rosemary, or basil.

Besides the salad you'll want a low-calorie protein: broiled chicken without the skin, or fish, veal, an omelette, or assorted low-fat cheeses. But no luncheon meats, with their many preservatives.

OUTWIT THE WAITER. Eating in restaurants calls for other strategies. Read only the top of the menu, where the intriguing appetizers are listed. Order one with negligible calories, such as a slice of melon or a shrimp cocktail. When it arrives, tell the waiter it looks so good that you'd like him to bring you yet a second appetizer. The second dish can be much higher in calories. Such departures from routine usually disconcert a busy establishment—so you'll surely be able to settle in for a fifteen- or twenty-minute wait before your second course finally arrives.

It's fun. You'll sample all sorts of piquant things you haven't eaten in years. But don't undo your good work by stumbling over the rolls and butter on your table. If you can afford the calories in something like a thin slice of pumpernickel toast, put that slice on your butter plate and ask the waiter to remove the tempting remainder.

Lunch over and you are still hungry? Look at your watch, know it takes some forty-five minutes for your body to register that you have eaten to satisfaction.

□ *DINNER*

This is the time for claiming your just rewards. It is the gold star for doing all that was expected of you throughout the day. It's certainly *not* the time to contend with a punishing diet. If the woman who prepares the meal can't eat it, the child within her is going to feel deprived. With no food to enjoy while her dinner partners are savoring theirs with gusto, she may pick at people. That's why I implore you to save 70 percent of your daily calories—875 of your 1,250—for a dinner you can approach with good-humored expectation.

On one of my lecture tours I remember spending a lovely day with a **very congenial woman**. I thought "Isn't she nice. I just wish she lived in San Diego so we could be friends." And then I had dinner at her home.

Perhaps because I was there, and had just delivered a talk about the importance of weight reduction, she had served herself hummingbird-sized portions of everything. And, perhaps because she felt denied, all she did throughout the entire meal was to pick at her children. At the end of twelve minutes, when the children stood up and said, "So long, Mom. So long, Pop. Gotta run," I felt like going too.

Dinner should be a cleverly staged ritual. By serving as many courses as you can contrive, one at a time, on as many appealing small dishes as you can assemble, you stretch out the presentation of food, dramatize the pleasure everyone extracts from it, and create an illusion of opulence. At The Golden Door I insist the waitresses give service that anywhere else would be considered terrible—attentive but poky. Each course comes at widespread intervals, and dessert never is served until at least forty-five minutes after we first sit down. All this ceremony makes a meal more satisfying. It improves conversation, too. I have never had a guest get up after dinner and say she was still hungry; the secret is in the forty-five minutes. Try it tonight!

Before the evening meal, serve an extravaganza of hors d'oeuvres, 50-

calorie raw vegetable snacks with a low-calorie dip. To accompany the *crudités,* add a champagne glass of something low-calorie and chilled, such as fruit juice over crushed ice, a wine spritzer, or a bit of champagne with orange juice.

Lastly—and with a flourish—serve dessert. Ripe fresh fruit, beautifully presented, or a frosty, fresh-fruit sherbet will satisfy your craving for sweets.

If you're single or alone for a while, switch luncheon and dinner by taking your main meal at noon. Celebrate it with a friend. Let dinner that evening be the simple salad and protein meal others had at lunch —who wants to eat a seven-course dinner alone?

□ *SIX WAYS TO CURTAIL CALORIES*

Here are six Golden Door techniques to help you cut weight sensibly and permanently:

1. SCHEDULE YOUR DELIGHTS. How you distribute your daily intake can be crucial to the success or failure of your food plan. Save your calories for the time of day you most need them—when they can give you the most pleasure, the most relaxation, and the most opportunity to communicate with someone else.

2. LET'S DECONTROL "PORTION CONTROL." Decorate your table with flowers and candles, not with food. Remember, no family-style "everything in the center of the table" platters. Serve only from the kitchen. If you do it properly, a five-year-old could tell which portion is intended for which person: the big portion to the person who wants to be bigger, and the small for whoever yearns to be smaller. Remember, garnishes both please and fool the eye, making portions seem larger. Pile on the parsley and mushrooms and lemon wedges.

3. EAT INEFFICIENTLY—PLAY WITH YOUR FOOD. Stretch out mealtimes for as long as possible, especially at dinner. Discard that well-remembered admonition from our childhood: "Don't play with your food."

Play with your food!

Why? Try inviting a thin friend for lunch. She'll pick at her plate, cut all her food into weird shapes, move it from the left side of the dish to the right, and only after a lot of handling will she put anything into her mouth. Then she will chew and chew. After your dish has been empty for five minutes, she might exclaim, "Oh! I'm keeping you waiting," and leave some of her food on the plate.

Then invite your fattest friend to luncheon and watch. You'll behold a model of efficiency. Cut, stab, lift, chew, all in a single motion. There goes one mouthful of food after another. She doesn't know it, but she might take in four times as much as the thin person does while performing the same amount of touching and chewing.

You know how this behavior originated. Mothers always applaud the quick, tidy eater faultlessly perched in the little high chair, each mouthful disappearing with no to-do. And they complain about the picky eater. There she sits, toying with her food, on and on for forty minutes while the exasperated mother could be doing other things. Today, the neat, tidy eater is on a diet. The picky eater is still a picky eater—and slender.

Teaching yourself to eat more slowly isn't easy, but once you recognize the necessity, you can find ways. Prove to yourself that a little food spread over a long time can be quite filling. Eat an entire meal with the aid of a junior-size set of utensils—not the little baby-size silver ones but the in-between size with the dull knife designed to protect children from cutting themselves. Or use a demitasse spoon and your smallest salad fork or cocktail fork. The little spoon probably won't make it through the consommé, and a good-sized salad will take forever to finish. You'll feel stuffed before dessert.

4. DECALORIZE. I borrowed the term "decalorize" from my friend Ruth West, who coined it in her splendid trend-setting cookbook, *Stop Dieting, Start Losing*. Ruth postulated that all your favorite recipes can remain intact as you craftily replace many high-calorie ingredients with low-calorie equivalents. Proceed in easy, sneaky steps over the months. By the time you've prepared and revised the dish ten or twelve times, nobody has noticed or kept track of the subtle change.

Most families have collected some treasured recipes they depend upon over and over. Write out your mainstay recipes even though you know them by heart. Then whenever you prepare one of them shave off 2 or 3 percent of the calories. Write down the amount you squeezed out.

Take spaghetti and meatballs as an example: Remove six strands of

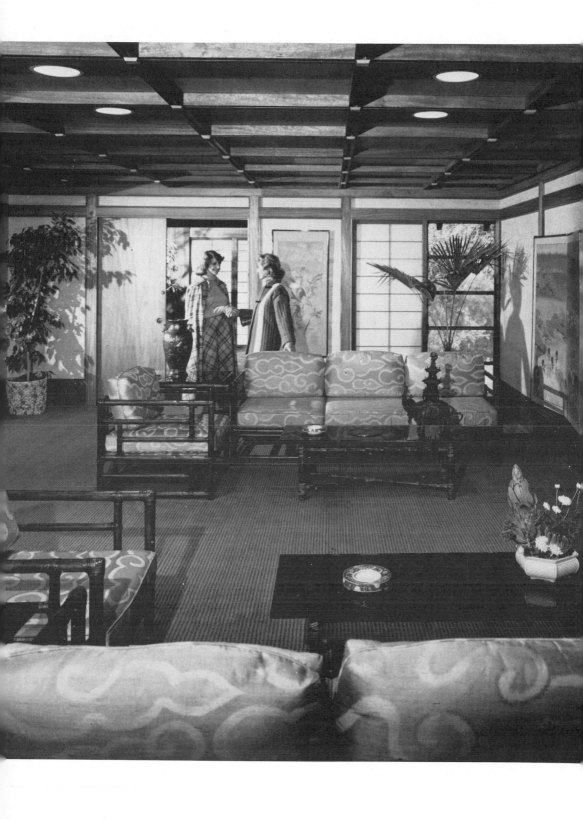

spaghetti and put six more mushrooms into the sauce. Next time, subtract six more strands and add a little eggplant with the mushrooms. The time after that, steal six more strands and increase the tomato. Soon your family will be dining contentedly on five or six ounces of spaghetti instead of eight.

Do the same thing with the meatballs. Instead of red meat only (four times the cholesterol, two to four times the calories, only half the protein of fish, chicken, veal, or cheese), introduce ground turkey, beans, or a soybean meal substitute. Then pad with a little more chopped onion, some chopped parsley, and a bit of grated carrot. On the day the meatball falls apart, you'll know you've gone too far. Backtrack, eliminating some of the carrot.

The same principle can be applied to all your favorite foods. It's especially effective for desserts, which can do nicely with 20 to 40 percent less sugar. Substitute fresh orange or other sweet fruit juice or purée for the sugar in that favorite cake. Work gradually. The sweet tooth can be weaned if you're patient.

The fact is that many people now are decalorizing without realizing it. Today, if you're serving ice cream and fruit, you'll probably pop a dollop of ice cream atop the fruit. A few years ago, there would have been a dab of fruit atop a mound of ice cream.

To get you started on your own system of decalorizing your favorite dishes, this chart suggests some lower-calorie substitutes for high-calorie standbys. (Calorie counts are given in parentheses.)

TRADITIONAL FOOD	CALORIE-SAVING FOOD	CALORIES SAVED
Apple pie, $\frac{1}{7}$ wedge of pie (350)	Baked apple (195)	155
Bacon, 2 slices fried crisp (100)	Canadian bacon, 2 slices (30)	70
Bagel, 1 (165)	Rye toast, 1 slice (60)	105
Beef, chuck, 4 ounces lean meat (180)	Beef round, 4 ounces lean meat (150)	30
Cheese, American, 1 ounce (105)	Mozzarella, 1 ounce (80)	25
Chicken, fried, 4 ounces (235)	Chicken, broiled, 4 ounces (150)	85
Chocolate cake, frosted, $\frac{1}{16}$ of cake (235)	Pound cake, $\frac{1}{2}$-inch slice (140)	95

TRADITIONAL FOOD	CALORIE-SAVING FOOD	CALORIES SAVED
Chocolate pudding, ½ cup (190)	Chocolate junket, ½ cup (120)	70
Clam chowder, New England, 1 cup (150)	Clam chowder, Manhattan, 1 cup (75)	75
Corn muffin, 1 medium (130)	Refrigerator biscuit, 1 (80)	50
Cream, light, 1 tablespoon (30)	Half-and-half, 1 tablespoon (20)	10
Cream of chicken soup, 1 cup (170)	Chicken noodle soup, 1 cup (65)	105
Egg, fried, 1 (110)	Egg, poached, soft- or hard-cooked, 1 (80)	30
English muffin, 1 (145)	Toast, 2 slices (120)	25
Fruit cocktail, canned, ½ cup (95)	Fruit salad, unsweetened refrigerated, ½ cup (55)	40
Grapefruit juice, sweetened, 1 cup (130)	Grapefruit juice, unsweetened, 1 cup (100)	30
Ice cream, 16% butterfat, 1 cup (375)	Ice cream, 10% butterfat, 1 cup (280)	95
Ice cream, 1 cup (280)	Ice milk, 1 cup (200)	80
Mayonnaise, 1 tablespoon (100)	Salad dressing, 1 tablespoon (65)	35
Milk, whole, 8 ounces (160)	Milk, skimmed, 8 ounces (90)	70
Orange juice, ½ cup (55)	Tomato juice, ½ cup (25)	30
Pecan pie, ⅐ of pie (490)	Pumpkin pie, ⅐ of pie (275)	215
Pineapple, canned, 1 slice, 2 tablespoons syrup (90)	Pineapple, canned in juice, 1 slice 2 tablespoons juice (70)	20
Potatoes, fried, homemade, 10 pieces (155)	Potatoes, fried from frozen, 10 pieces (125)	30
Potato chips, 10 medium (115)	Popcorn, buttered, 1 cup (40)	75
Pudding, vanilla, from whole milk, 1 cup (275)	Pudding, vanilla, from skimmed milk, 1 cup (205)	70
Quinine water, 8 ounces (85)	Club soda, 8 ounces (0)	85
Ricotta cheese, ½ cup (170)	Cottage cheese, creamed, ½ cup (120)	50
Salad oil (used in cooking), 1 tablespoon (125)	Butter or margarine (used in cooking), 1 tablespoon (100)	25
Salmon, canned sockeye, 4 ounces (200)	Salmon, canned pink or chum, 4 ounces (160)	40
Strawberry shortcake, 1 serving with whipped cream (465)	Strawberries in dry wine, 1 serving (100)	365

TRADITIONAL FOOD	CALORIE-SAVING FOOD	CALORIES SAVED
Sweet potatoes, candied, ½ cup (295)	Winter squash, buttered, ½ cup (95)	200
Whipped cream, homemade, 1 tablespoon (30)	Whipped cream, from aerosol, 1 tablespoon (10)	20
Yogurt, strawberry flavor, 8-ounce container (290)	Yogurt, vanilla flavor, 8-ounce container (220)	70

Food writers in the United States have been according a lot of space to a "new" French cuisine that emphasizes clean, lean crispness without all the fattening sauces considered de rigueur by the old Escoffier school of French chefs. A Washington reporter friend who follows such things thinks the French simply are catching on to a style of cookery that we have been practicing in America for some time.

So-called "soft" drinks are never served at The Golden Door—not even the sugar-free diet kind. Nor will I allow them in my home. I was dismayed to read a survey released by *Advertising Age* which disclosed that Americans are now guzzling more pop than coffee, formerly the number-one beverage. According to the survey, the per capita figure for last year was a whopping 34.8 gallons for each of us. Whatever happened to drinking a glass of water when thirsty?

5. STAY AWARE.   Look at your plate and learn how to gauge what is on it; correlate it with what you have eaten and what you will eat ("It's lunch now. What did I eat for breakfast, and what will I be having for dinner?"). Before each meal, ask yourself, "What have I already done today, what am I about to do?" Eat accordingly. A day of driving, telephoning, and desk work suggests a light breakfast and luncheon. But if this is the day you're playing four sets of tennis you can say, "Aha! I deserve an extra piece of toast! I've earned it!"

6. HOW TO SURVIVE A COCKTAIL PARTY.   One of the bonuses of new vitality is that you'll be finding time for all the tempting social invitations sent you, and you'll receive more of them. One of the drawbacks is that you'll wend your way again and again to that fattening tribal gathering, the cocktail party.

Before leaving your home, raise your blood-sugar level so you won't be too famished when you arrive at the party. Slice yourself a big piece of melon, or prepare a dish of strawberries or a salad. If you're short of time, take along some sliced raw vegetables to nibble in the car.

If the invitation reads six-thirty, make your entrance at seven-fifteen. This has nothing to do with fashionable lateness; it's just that by seven-thirty or so the hors d'oeuvres will have been picked over, saving you from tantalizing temptations. Also, you'll have time for no more than two drinks, maximum, before dinner.

Once you've joined the party, if you're anything like me, you should locate the peanuts in order to decide the part of the room you're not going to be in. It's simpler to avoid them. And never station yourself within reach of the hors d'oeuvres or the buffet table. Make certain to be as far from it as you can.

Now for the heart of the matter—the cocktail itself. In Washington, D.C., the cocktail party is absolutely a way of life, so I was startled to hear a friend there say she's managed to switch completely away from hard liquor.

"I haven't had a drop for three years because I remember you saying three ounces of wine costs us the same number of calories as an ounce of hard liquor. I never cared much about liquor anyway. The only thing I drink now is wine—usually in the form of a spritzer, because soda water makes it go even farther." This is no longer the exception; it is the rule.

If you don't want to wrench yourself from a lifetime of martinis to one of white-wine spritzers, start weaning yourself by asking for a tall glass of club soda with lime when you arrive at a party. It will quench your thirst. Then have your first alcoholic drink. After that, if you still want something to sip, have another club soda with lime, alternating in this fashion till dinnertime.

□ THE ESSENCE OF GOOD NUTRITION: QUALITY IN YOUR FOOD

So far, you've covered just two elements of a three-hundred-sixty-five-day health horoscope: First, how to balance energy intake with energy output (remember, the iron law of calorie control is the same as the First Law of Thermodynamics: a definite amount of heat can be converted into a definite amount of energy) and, second, some very logical ways to augment the sheer satisfaction of eating. The missing third element is, of course, good nutrition.

The next time you look at the "enrichments" and additives listed on a food container, reflect for a moment on what standards you have a right to set for your body's fuel. And then ask yourself what was removed from the product to make some of those additives necessary. Think for a moment. Where do the preservatives go? You're mistaken if you suppose these chemicals will preserve you.

Barbra Streisand ended a lifelong affair with junk foods during a week at The Golden Door, without anything like the struggle she thought she would endure:

> I was so sure I was going to feel deprived that, before I went, I stocked up on hot dogs and Cokes . . . but it was wonderful, and my skin was as clear as a bell. It isn't a radical thing with me—the food there was organic, but it doesn't have to be. . . . Just eat good healthful food. The point is, if you know that what you're putting into your system is good, it makes you feel good about yourself.

□ WAYS TO ENSURE QUALITY IN YOUR FOOD

1. Eat the freshest fruits and vegetables; if possible, grow a small garden.
2. Select the most natural unprocessed foods (those without additives or preservatives).

3. Remember, cholesterol is a chancy fat. Ongoing research constantly produces new information, so do read your newspapers and magazines to keep up-to-date—then use your common sense.
4. Avoid sugar and salt; use very, *very* cautiously and only occasionally.
5. Look to the quality of water.

1. THE FRESHEST FRUITS AND VEGETABLES.   I once read a U. S. Department of Agriculture pamphlet that traced the vitamin C content of a head of lettuce traveling from field to market to restaurant. This particular head lost 85 percent of its vitamin C before it reached a salad bowl. Food on most family tables is not fresh. Oddly enough, the offender here isn't The System—it's the American housewife.

Here's what happens in many cities. That head of lettuce is picked and rushed to a nearby packinghouse where the outer leaves are removed; the lettuce is washed, crated, and flung onto a truck. That very night the truck rushes down the highway and arrives in a produce market at two in the morning. At four, your local supermarket picks up the lettuce and at six a shift goes on to set out the fresh produce.

Later that day the efficient American housewife drops by with her weekly shopping list. It says she needs three heads of lettuce. Into her shopping cart they go, to languish in her refrigerator for many days. Also on her list are string beans and carrots. In they go with her weekly purchases, although the green string beans look yellow and limp, and she could have taken home fresh, sleek, shiny eggplant.

Ideally, we all should live by Confucius' dictum about diet: Eat nothing but fresh food, in season, locally grown. Obviously, we can't. But 80 percent out of a hundred wouldn't be bad. In the average supermarket you're offered numerous choices. Treat yourself to nothing but the best foodstuffs. You will find them more affordable once you begin to shop every second day and for the exact number of people you will be feeding, as well as the appropriate amount each person requires. Select foods that stir your senses. Shop with eyes and tactile senses alert for the most bedazzling colors, scents, and textures. It's one way to determine how close your food is to its natural state, straight out of the earth or off a tree. Food which provides this kind of sensory satisfaction has a better chance of providing the Total Calorie all of us need.

Once I visited Paris when the children were small, and because I wanted babysitters we stayed at a small *pension*-like hotel. There was no menu choice. We ate what was put before us. Since we usually lunched at different restaurants, I would ask the cook what she planned for dinner so we wouldn't eat the same thing two meals in a row. On the third day she slammed down a pot, whirled on me with her arms waving, and screamed, "How can I know what will leap into my market basket?"

She shopped daily—with an empty basket, an almost-empty purse, and an open mind. She bought what was in season, freshest, and best. So should we.

2. SELECT THE MOST NATURAL FOODS. Always remember that we, too, are part of nature; we do best with that which is closest to nature. I'm not advocating moving to a cabbage patch, but I'm a great believer in home gardens, whenever and wherever possible. The advantages stretch beyond the realm of nutrition and touch on every aspect of the Total Calorie.

Puttering in a vegetable garden is one of the finest of exercises. Physically, it provides caloric expenditure and a vast array of sensory diversions. Psychologically, it can transform the most meager salad into an object of infinite pride and satisfaction.

Another bell-ringing bonus: fresh fruits and vegetables require minimal cooking time. Just add a bit of water or a few lettuce leaves to them in a tightly sealed, heavy pan (not aluminum). No need for sauces or strong seasonings, which only interfere with texture and color.

Simplicity is the keynote. There's a world of difference between a teaspoon of cornflakes and a bite out of a fresh ear of corn. Beware of processing, which in food means to add, subtract, modify, and transform.

I've always devoutly believed in the dietary worth of fibers, raw vegetables, and whole grains. Recent research has exposed links between diseases of civilization—certain forms of cancer, appendicitis, varicose veins, phlebitis, diabetes, ischemic heart disease—and the roller-milling which replaced the fiber-preserving stone-grinding of earlier centuries.

When you next go to market, play this game to reinforce your new convictions. Choose the longest line at the checkout stand. Peer closely at the contents of each cart and scrutinize the person behind it. I'll bet the cart piled highest with boxes and cans, six-packs of pop, frozen foods and cookies, potato chips, and loaves of white bread has behind it the harried-looking, washed-out, old-in-her-thirties woman you've seen in the line many times and scarcely noticed. If you see a cart stacked with fresh vegetables and fruits, cornucopia-like with greens and yellows and reds and browns, I'll be surprised if the person pushing it doesn't appear happy and healthy. Then look at your own cart. Think "Here is my energy, my family's energy."

3. CHOLESTEROL IS A CHANCY FAT. Most of what you read about cholesterol is true. The human body needs and manufactures cholesterol, yet in excess it is dangerous.

It may not be *as* dangerous by itself as doctors a few years ago were saying it was. Sugar now is suspected of as much guilt in the matter of heart attacks. But cholesterol still is something to be wary of. There are dozens of available books and medical journals describing cholesterol and how it affects us when ingested in excess, so be on the lookout for the most up-to-date information.

Keep in mind too that food, whether it's carbohydrates, protein, or fat, when not used for energy must be stored as fat or it may be used for making cholesterol. Either way surplus fat storage is weighty and the potential for dis-ease.

Many pediatricians advise skim milk or low-fat milk for newborns. Technically, everybody begins to die at the first breath of life. But aging and the symptoms of senility are definitely accelerated by the shadow of cholesterol which lines our arteries. Middle-aged and older men, as well as postmenopausal women, run the highest risk of heart attack. Even if nothing traumatic happens, the overall efficiency of the body suffers.

Americans used to believe this country's much-vaunted standard of living dictated large amounts of steaks, lamb, pork, dairy products, and other animal fats. These contain "saturated" fats, the ones that elevate blood lipids, in contrast to "polyunsaturated" fats found in vegetable products like safflower oil and corn oil, which actually tend to lower blood lipids.

If you're planning to lose weight, you'll be interested in a theory that people who yo-yo up and down the scales are setting themselves up as high-risk targets. At such times it's of importance to stay with the foods low in saturated fats.

You can reduce the amount of cholesterol and other saturated fats you ingest by limiting your consumption of dairy products. Reserve breakfast eggs for Saturday or Sunday brunch, and on those days avoid eggs in your lunch or dinner. If your physician advises caution, whip up omelets or soufflés using one egg yolk to two egg whites, thereby cutting your cholesterol by 50 percent. I don't like any of the egg substitutes; read the list of their ingredients, and you'll see why.

When buying cheese, look for some of the fine skim-milk and semi-skim-milk cheeses. You don't have to give up your favorite whole-milk cheeses altogether. Just allow yourself two of the semi-skim-milk cheeses for one of the whole-milk variety. A useful if not exact rule to gauge fat content: the harder the cheese, the lower in fat it's likely to be.

Twice a week should be maximum for red meat. Save it for special occasions. Also be very cautious about organs; liver, kidneys, and sweet-breads are loaded with cholesterol.

Use polyunsaturated oils. If you're purchasing margarine, read the package label to be positive the product you're buying consists of 100 percent liquid corn oil. Look for the same quality—100 percent poly-unsaturated—in salad oils (preferably corn, sesame, and safflower). If you are extremely fond of olive oil, as I am, then blend one-half olive with one-half corn oil. You will like it even better.

4. AVOID EXCESS SUGAR AND SALT.   Many doctors concede that choles-terol buildup may not be a major inducer of heart attacks, but just an indication of something going wrong. Instead, they're beginning to look critically at that seemingly innocuous box of sugar on your shelf.

Most people are unaware that they eat about one hundred pounds of sugar a year, since so much of it lurks in processed foods, says Dr. John Yudkin, formerly Professor of Nutrition at the University of London, and a crusader against sugar. Some of the other points he makes:

a. The old adage that sugar gives you more energy than other foods is phony. Energy is another word for calories, and you can get them from any food.

b. Natural sugar, from raw fruits and unprocessed vegetables, is perfectly all right. You can't eat enough to overdose on it since it's in combination with its host fruit, which contains all the proper proportions of minerals, vitamins, and enzymes.

c. Refined sugar is a poison in the doses many people take of it. Lives are being shortened by unwise eating habits.

Excess salt, like sugar, is bad for you. Its effects are cumulative, and as little as three grams a day (about a teaspoon) contributes to hypertension. Americans consume far too much salt. Learn finesse in the use of seasonings like herbs, spices, and puréed vegetables—all of which can substitute for salt.

5. LOOK TO THE QUALITY OF WATER. Pure fresh water is a primary consideration. Your body itself is composed chiefly of water. For both drinking and cooking, obtain good spring water with all trace minerals intact. If you don't have satisfactory local springs, investigate some stellar names among the world's bottled mineral waters.

Do drink the recommended six to eight glasses of water each day, always between meals, never with. You can flavor it with freshly squeezed lemon juice if you wish. I like to picture my insides being washed just as much as I anticipate a shower.

□ *THE PLUS AND MINUS WAY TO BALANCE YOUR WEIGHT*

When I had to come up with a plan to help a busy executive follow a weight-loss program and still accommodate business luncheons, cocktails, and dinner engagements, I created a technique you may find helpful too.

It's a system of balances: pluses and minuses. Starting tomorrow, spend a minute each day grading yourself on the previous day. Enter on your calendar a plus if you ate too much; a minus if you were an angel and ordered yogurt and fruit for lunch and fish and a vegetable for dinner; and a zero for the day you neither lost nor gained.

You'll quickly become very handy at setting up a couple of days of compensatory minuses when you intend to dine well on Friday, Saturday, or Sunday. In the same way you'll become quietly proficient at squeezing in an extra hour of exercise that might balance your food intake.

On Monday, review the week past. If you earn one extra minus a week, you most likely have achieved for yourself a laudable deficit of about 875 calories. Four such weeks a month can mean a loss of one pound of fat.

A man using the system can now join in decision-making in which he otherwise was merely a bystander. Contemplating a coming day in which he has a business luncheon and his wife has a board-meeting, he may say to her, "My love, let's both order cottage cheese and salad for lunch. Then let's have eggplant and fish for dinner tonight—there's no way we can keep tomorrow from being a plus." What is so revolutionary about this simple system—and has made it a watchword among Golden Door guests—is that it involves both partners, many for the first time, in determining what they eat.

KNOW THYSELF. Here is an important perception that The Golden Door teaches as it modifies your attitudes toward food:

Each time you regard any dish of food set before you, pause a moment, think, say if you like, "This is me, my vitality, my body, the fuel for my day." See the food as units of energy hopping all over the plate— "This part I will use during my exercise, this part for sitting at my desk, this part for sleeping, and oh! do I want to store this or leave it on my plate?"

□ THE VIRTUE-MAKING DAY— BETTER THAN FASTING

Perhaps you're feeling heavy and stale after a party weekend or a long stretch of sedentary work. Maybe you'd like to drop a few pounds. If so, try the Virtue-Making Day (so called by the first guests who ever tried it because it made them feel so saintly), which almost all guests follow for one day at The Door and then take home.

This plan is so much more comforting than a day of fasting; because you have continuous blood-sugar builders, you should feel neither hungry nor weak; and there's no chance of loss of body tissue.

□ *DIET FOR THE GOLDEN DOOR*
VIRTUE-MAKING DAY

(Note: with the exception of almond milk, with each serving
of liquid eat ½ ounce sunflower seeds and 3 pine nuts.)

8:00 A.M. GRAPEFRUIT JUICE
4 oz. freshly squeezed grapefruit juice
2 oz. water
Mix and serve.

10:30 A.M. ALMOND MILK
6 whole almonds, blanched and peeled
½ medium-sized ripe banana
½ cup water
2 ice cubes
few drops fresh lemon juice
dash of vanilla
dash of nutmeg
Place in blender, liquefy, and serve.

1:00 P.M. GAZPACHO
1 medium tomato, peeled and diced
¼ large cucumber, peeled and chopped
¼ large green pepper, seeded and chopped
1 onion slice
2 sprigs parsley
Place in blender, liquefy, and serve.

3:30 P.M. PINEAPPLE-CUCUMBER JUICE
3 oz. cucumber, peeled
1 oz. fresh pineapple
2 sprigs parsley
2 oz. apple juice
Place in blender, liquefy, and serve.

6:00 P.M. ALMOND MILK

8:30 P.M. CARROT-APPLE JUICE
2 oz. apple juice
2 oz. carrot juice
⅓ apple, peeled
Place in blender, liquefy, and serve.

□ NOTES FOR THE VIRTUE-MAKING DIET

This regimen is recommended for people in average good health but is not advised for those troubled by diabetes, hypoglycemia, or any condition requiring medical care. Do check with your physician if you have any doubts.

1. No to coffee and tea. Yes to freshly squeezed, unsweetened lemonade, herb teas, and spring water—as much and as often as you please.
2. You must consume liquids slowly, using a demitasse spoon. Nibble (just as slowly) on the sunflower seeds, which should be hulled, raw, and unsalted. Chew them one by one, with distinct relish.
3. Before each mini-meal, or juice break, step outdoors, even if it's snowing. Breathe consciously. About twenty times, inhale deeply and exhale very, very slowly and thoroughly. Imagine a total oxygen exchange throughout your mind/body. Remain aware of your mind/body as you return to your day.

You will find this day so much more comfortable and comforting than a day of fasting, because you have continuous blood-sugar builders every two and a half hours—a juice break providing diversion and sustaining resolve. You should feel neither hungry, weak, nor tense.

□ WHY VEGETARIANISM?

If vegetarianism is your thing, as it is mine, you'll find medical research increasingly supportive.

> Macrobiotic vegetarians, checked against people who were quite similar except for being nonvegetarian, have lower blood pressure and leaner bodies. Now a scientific team in Boston has reported that a commune-based vegetarian group, carefully studied and tested, showed significantly lower blood cholesterol and triglyceride levels—important factors associated with lower risk of heart attack.
>
> The research team, from Boston City Hospital and Harvard Medical School, measured the blood lipids, or fats, in 116 vegetarians whose diets

consisted of whole grains, beans, fresh vegetables, seaweed, and fermented soy products. For additional foods, the vegetarians like fruits, nuts, beer, and fish. Some eat dairy foods; a few eat eggs. These subjects were matched for age and sex with nonvegetarians on the usual American diet. Blood-fat scores were found strikingly low in the vegetarians, who had only slight rises with increased age. Eating dairy foods and eggs increased the lipid scores; but fish, though eaten more often, had no effect on cholesterol or triglyceride levels.

One vegetarian, found to have an abnormal cholesterol condition, was the source of important clues. During a few weeks when he was off the macrobiotic diet, his plasma lipids jumped up; when he was back on the diet, the lipid levels quickly settled back.

The study team, reporting its findings in *The New England Journal of Medicine,* includes scientist Frank M. Sacks, Dr. William Castelli, Allen Donner, Ph.D., and Dr. Edward Kass. They believe the health values of the vegetarian diet deserve further research. Vegetarianism could be good medicine for patients with special blood lipid problems.

CHAPTER VII

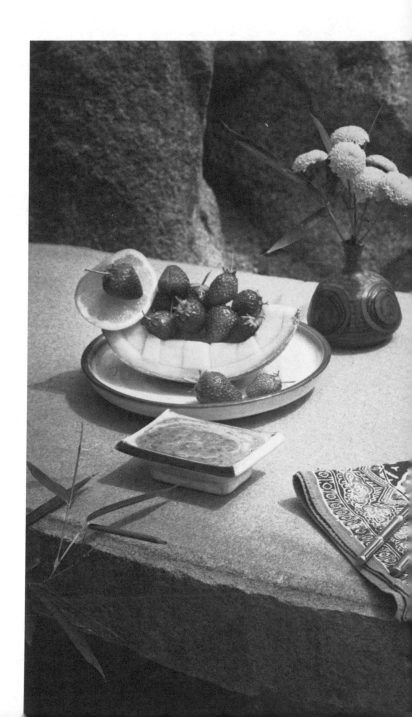

THE
GOLDEN DOOR
MENUS

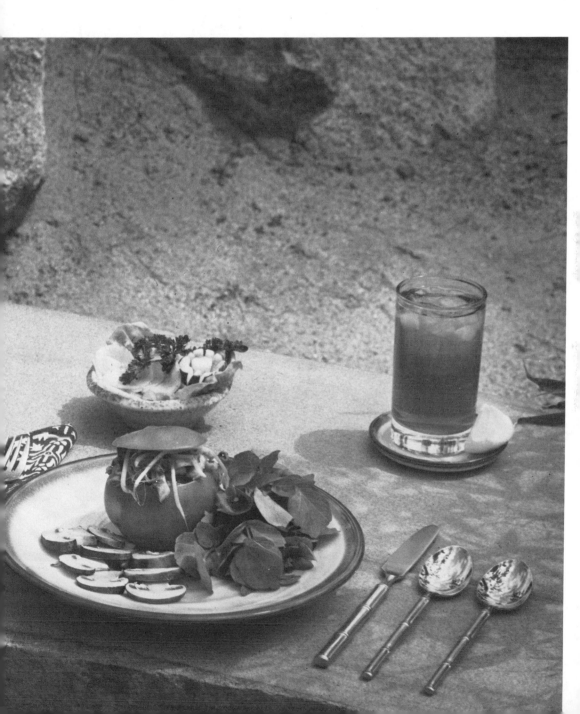

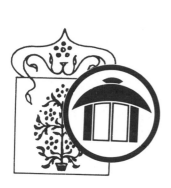

□ INTRODUCING THE
GOLDEN DOOR MENUS

Y EARS AGO, I SPENT MANY EXHAUSTING HOURS IN THE KITCHEN
at Rancho La Puerta preparing meals for our early guests.
Daily I ground wheat, baked bread, milked goats and made
cheese, rinsed sprouts, nursed our acidophilus-milk culture,
and grew, canned, and even dried in the sun a great assortment of vegetables and fruits.

My guests of today are being served with every bit as much pride,
but far less effort. The superb and simple Golden Door food, in the
opinion of many, is my spa's most outstanding claim to fame. It antici-
pated by many years the *cuisine minceur* of present-day French chefs.

Now my time in food preparation has been reduced to an occasional
precious and privileged hour in my own kitchen on a quiet Sunday.
But in my fancy I never really have left the kitchen. I still invade the

211

delicious territory of my cookbook shelf—I feel that if a recipe cannot in itself arouse my taste buds, it isn't worth cooking.

The following menus and recipes are selected from the hundreds of favorites served at The Golden Door. They represent one full month—four weeks of tantalizing, satisfying food, planned to help you normalize your weight. As you turn the pages, try to smell, savor, and visualize these popular Golden Door dishes. Remember, they are all the more delectable because almost every ingredient is fresh and unprocessed.

In assembling the menus and recipes, I've tried to create an eating plan that can gracefully be adapted to many life-styles. I've chosen menus that will fit easily into your eating patterns—meals that are varied, quick, and enjoyable to prepare, yet satisfying at your dinner table.

It would be preposterous to try to create the perfect diet for the average person. There is no perfect diet. And, as I have said before, there is no average person. Use the following meals and recipes as a loose frame for you to adjust and readjust around the shifting elements of your everyday life.

Each recipe is low in calories, but all calorie counts are necessarily approximate—for the size and even the quality of an ingredient will affect the total calorie content.

There are twenty-eight menus in all; four groups of seven each compose a hypothetical week. In each group, five of the menus are arranged as dinners for two. If you are cooking for more than two who wish to lose weight, you can easily multiply the ingredients. Each week of menus also contains a low-calorie entertainment dinner for six. Completing the selection is a brunch or late, light supper. Most of the meals can be prepared in thirty to forty minutes, with the exception of the international and entertainment recipes, which you should be able to put together in about an hour.

The dressings and sauces all were developed at The Golden Door and are significantly reduced in calories. They can be prepared ahead and refrigerated or frozen in small portions to be used as required in many of the recipes. You will note that little or no salt is used in these sauces. Almost all Americans salt their food much too heavily, and for that reason I recommend going light on salt, heavy on herbs and spices

—with an ever-vigilant emphasis on fresh ingredients which have undergone the least possible amount of processing. If your doctor has recommended a salt-free diet, increase the herbs and spices, and cut out the salt entirely: You won't miss it.

The only special equipment you will need is a food blender (liquefier). If you are short on time, you will discover that the Cuisinart, or one of its competitors, does so much more than blend or chop or liquefy; it is an extraordinary substitute for one more pair of hands. Whichever you employ, an instant sauce or dressing can be made by blending a piece of cooked vegetable with the juices in which it was cooked and adding a few simple herbs as seasoning. An elegant dessert can be concocted from a slice of really ripe fruit served in a pretty dish and topped with another liquefied fruit of contrasting flavor and color.

I have not included recipes for breakfast or luncheon. Please see pages 186–189 for suggestions and for the vital discussion of caloric apportionment.

The best way to utilize these menus effectively is to choose the one that matches your caloric need for the day. For instance, if you overeat at luncheon, choose the dinner menu with the lowest calorie count. The five varied dinner menus for two offer you many options: one is very low-calorie, one is vegetarian, one is international, one is Golden Door gourmet, and one is a quickie.

If one serving is not sufficient because you have a greater caloric need, there are several alternatives: increase the portion size; add a slice of Tecate Bread (page 279) or a starch such as a potato; include a serving of whole grains like bulgur wheat, brown rice, or buckwheat groats. Or take an afternoon pick-me-up such as a wedge of cheese and a piece of fruit. Or eat more at breakfast and/or luncheon. And remember that portion size should never be dictated by dollars and cents, but according to the pounds and inches of the person being served.

Weight loss should be sensible, steady, and slow, so that vitality will be enhanced and in no way diminished.

Above all, bear in mind that the most important ingredient you can add to a meal is joy. (And, before you turn to the menus and recipes, I want to express thanks for the joyous contribution of Michel Stroot, the best chef The Golden Door has ever had.)

☐ **WEEK I OF DINNER MENUS**
FOR WEIGHT REDUCTION

		CALORIES
1 Very low cal	WATERCRESS SALAD MUSHROOM SOUFFLÉ BANANA-ORANGE CRUNCH	60 265 180
	TOTAL:	505
2 Vegetarian	GARDEN SOUP EGGPLANT PARMESAN FRUTTO VINO	55 435 115
	TOTAL:	605
3 International	MIDDLE-EASTERN ANISE BREW WORRY-BEAD APPETIZER FISH KEBABS SHREDDED VEGETABLE SALAD BROILED GRAPEFRUIT	75 250 115 65
	TOTAL:	505
4 Golden Door Gourmet	OLIVE-STUFFED ARTICHOKES CHICKEN CHASSEUR ZUCCHINI FORMAGGIO NAVEL ORANGE	25 220 195 75
	TOTAL:	515
5 Quickie	1 SLICE TECATE BREAD, TOASTED TURKEY SALAD DIVAN CARAMEL CUSTARD	100 270 205
	TOTAL:	575
6 Brunch or late, late supper	ZUCCHINI SALAD ANDALOUSE PAUPIETTE OF VEAL ROULATINE CREAM OF MANGO AU KIWI	50 400 100
	TOTAL:	550

WHITE-WINE SPRITZER	45
PEASANT CAVIAR	85
GOLDEN DOOR BREAST OF CHICKEN	310
GARDEN OF VEGETABLES	110
APPIAN PEARS	175
TOTAL:	725

VERY LOW CAL

WATERCRESS SALAD

(Each serving, 60 calories)

The quality of this salad depends on the absolute freshness of the watercress. Spinach and curly endive, mixed half and half, may be substituted if watercress is not available.

½ large tomato, peeled and diced
¼ teaspoon Golden Door seasoning salt (see page 277)
¼ teaspoon freshly ground pepper
1 tablespoon Golden Door vinaigrette dressing (see dressing for Golden Door Combination Salad, page 243)
1 bunch watercress
1 to 2 ounces fresh bean sprouts
1 teaspoon chopped chives or scallions
1 tablespoon sunflower seeds

Season the tomato and pour the dressing over it. Wash the watercress and remove the stems. Just before serving, add the bean sprouts to the tomato and watercress. Sprinkle with chives and toss. Add the sunflower seeds and toss again. Serve immediately.

MUSHROOM SOUFFLE

(Each serving, 265 calories)

1 tablespoon plus 1 teaspoon 100% corn-oil margarine
2 cups finely chopped fresh mushrooms (about ⅓ pound)
¼ cup finely chopped mild onion (Bermuda or green onion, or shallot)
1 very small clove garlic, minced
4 teaspoons unbleached flour
salt, pepper, and nutmeg
2 teaspoons lemon juice
2 tablespoons white wine, milk, or water
3 eggs, at room temperature, separated

Melt 1 tablespoon margarine in frying pan over high heat. Add mushrooms, onion, and garlic. Cook, stirring, until mixture begins to brown and most of the moisture has gone. Remove from heat. Sprinkle with flour, ¼ teaspoon salt, pepper, and a dash of nutmeg. Stir to coat evenly. Add lemon juice and wine, cool, then blend in egg yolks.

Preheat oven to 375° F. Grease 2 soufflé dishes of 1½- to 2-cup capacity with as little margarine as possible.

Beat egg whites with ⅛ teaspoon salt until they hold peaks but still look moist. Fold (don't stir) half the whites into mushrooms until fully blended. Partially fold in remaining whites. Immediately pour into dishes and bake about 15 to 18 minutes, or until centers no longer feel liquid when gently touched. Eat at once. (A soufflé falls less rapidly if served on hot plates and spooned from the outside, not the center.)

BANANA-ORANGE CRUNCH

Each serving, 180 calories)

1 medium banana, peeled and sliced

¼ cup fresh or canned mandarin oranges, drained

1 teaspoon honey

1 teaspoon lemon juice

2 tablespoons fine graham-cracker crumbs

1 tablespoon chopped nuts

1 tablespoon 100% corn-oil margarine

Combine banana, oranges, honey, and lemon juice in a bowl and chill. Sauté crumbs and nuts in the margarine over low heat until crumbs are toasted. Place fruit mixture in two dessert dishes and sprinkle with crumbs.

Note: You may substitute any favorite fruit for the mandarin oranges.

VEGETARIAN

GARDEN SOUP

(Each serving, 55 calories)

2 cups chicken broth (see page 278)

1 carrot, sliced ¼-inch thick

2 green onions, including part of green tops, sliced (reserve remaining green tops)

½ cup raw green beans, cut into 1-inch pieces, or broccoli flowerettes

½ green or red bell pepper, diced

salt and pepper

Heat chicken broth, add vegetables, and simmer about 5 to 10 minutes, or until vegetables are tender-crisp. About 2 minutes before serving, add reserved green onion tops and season with salt and pepper.

EGGPLANT PARMESAN
(Each serving, 435 calories)

Make the tomato sauce first and then proceed with the recipe. See the recipe for Tomato Sauce (page 278) or use this recipe:

1 (8-ounce) can tomato sauce	¼ teaspoon anise or fennel seed
1 large clove garlic, puréed	(optional)
⅛ teaspoon each dried basil and oregano	

In small sauce pan combine all ingredients. Bring to boil and simmer for 20 minutes, stirring occasionally.

4 slices unpeeled eggplant, ½-inch thick	1 tablespoon minced fresh parsley
½ cup nonfat milk	salt and pepper
2 tablespoons unbleached flour	2 tablespoons olive oil (approximate)
1 egg	2 ounces Swiss or Monterey Jack cheese, cut into 2 slices
1 tablespoon water	sprinkle of grated Parmesan cheese
1 green onion with part of green top, minced	tomato sauce

Salt eggplant, marinate in milk for 10 minutes, remove, and pat dry (discard milk).

Put flour on a plate. In bowl wide enough to hold eggplant, blend egg, water, green onion, parsley, salt and pepper to taste. Heat 1 tablespoon oil in large frying pan over medium heat.

Dip each eggplant slice in flour to coat, then in egg mixture. Fry slowly until golden brown. Turn, adding rest of oil to brown other side. Eggplant should be nearly tender when finished. Cool slightly.

Place 1 slice eggplant and 1 slice cheese into individual baking dishes. Top with a second eggplant slice. Smother each with tomato sauce and top with grated Parmesan cheese.

Bake at 375° F. until hot and bubbly (15 minutes if all ingredients are warm when assembled) .

FRUTTO VINO
(Each serving, 115 calories)

⅓ cup sherry   1 apple
1 orange

Heat wine just until it starts to simmer, to reduce alcoholic calories. Cool.

Peel orange; remove as much white membrane as possible; slice thinly and remove seeds. Core unpeeled apple, slice thinly, and coat with some juice from the orange to prevent discoloration. Pour wine over fruit and chill, turning once to marinate, about 15 minutes. Serve with slices arranged alternately in bowl with marinade.

INTERNATIONAL
MIDDLE-EASTERN ANISE BREW
(Each serving, 75 calories)

The favorite alcoholic drink all over the Near and Middle East is a clear anise-flavored brew that turns milky when water or ice is added. The Greeks call it ouzo; the Turks, raki; and the Arabs, arrack. This recipe duplicates the flavor.

¼ teaspoon anise extract   6 ice cubes, cracked or crushed
¼ cup very dry white wine

Add extract to wine and stir. Serve over cracked ice.

WORRY-BEAD APPETIZER

Throughout the Middle East, people finger strings of "worry beads" to relieve tension. Unfortunately, it is possible to fiddle with the beads single-handedly, leaving the other hand free for food, drink, and nicotine.

Cracking *unshelled* sunflower seeds, also a Middle Eastern pastime, serves the purpose better than beads. It occupies both hands. Also, the seeds are so tiny and troublesome to get at that it is almost impossible to overeat.

A sunflower-seed researcher armed with calorie-count book, scale, clock, and basic arithmetic produced these startling findings: It took nearly 30 minutes to crack ⅓ cup (or 175 seeds), which weighed ⅓ ounce and had a total calorie count of about 55.

Conclusion: Crack all the sunflower seeds you have patience for, and eat them as an appetizer with your drink before dinner.

FISH KEBABS
(Each serving, 250 calories)

1 tablespoon olive oil	1 lemon
⅔ pound very firm fish, cut into 1-inch cubes	8 bay leaves, broken in half

Sprinkle 1 teaspoon oil over fish. Cut lemon in half and squeeze juice of one half onto fish. Add bay leaves and toss to coat. Marinate for about 15 minutes.

Cut remaining lemon half, including rind, into ¾-inch wedges. Heat remaining 2 teaspoons oil in large frying pan over medium-high heat. Add lemon wedges, cover until spattering dies down, uncover, and sauté until glazed and golden brown. Remove and cool.

Thread 4 to 6 short skewers alternately with fish, lemon wedges, and bay leaves. Broil skewers, turning to brown all sides. Fish is done when no longer translucent inside. Total cooking time should be about 5 to 6 minutes. The charring of bay leaves and lemon is desirable—it contributes delightful flavor.

SHREDDED VEGETABLE SALAD
(Each serving, 115 calories)

The white radish (*beyaz turp*) used in this Turkish salad is the same mild, foot-long type found here in Oriental grocery stores and many supermarkets. Its Japanese name is *daikon;* the Chinese name is *loh bok.*

If you can't find the radish, just make the salad with carrot and cabbage and garnish it with red radishes. Or substitute shredded turnip or raw beet.

lettuce leaves
2 carrots, shredded
1 cup shredded green or red
cabbage

1 cup shredded mild white radish
1 tablespoon olive oil
4 pickled peppers (*peperoncino*)
1 lemon, cut into 4 wedges

Line salad plates with lettuce. Toss each shredded vegetable separately with 1 teaspoon oil. On each plate arrange a tricolored mound of the three separate vegetables. Garnish each plate with 2 peppers and 2 lemon wedges. Squeeze lemon juice over salad before eating.

BROILED GRAPEFRUIT

(Each serving, 65 calories)

1 grapefruit, preferably pink
2 teaspoons brown sugar

pinch of ground ginger
2 fresh strawberries, cut in half

Cut grapefruit in half; cut out membrane in center and loosen segments with knife. Sprinkle with sugar and ginger. Place in a baking pan and bake at 375° F. for 15 minutes, or until very hot and bubbly. Put berries in centers. Serve hot.

GOLDEN DOOR GOURMET

OLIVE-STUFFED ARTICHOKES

(Each serving, 25 calories)

If you use fresh cooked artichokes to prepare this, save the leaves with edible tips. Squeeze lemon juice over them and use some for garnish. The rest can be refrigerated for a low-calorie snack or salad.

2 anchovy fillets, minced
(optional)
½ teaspoon drained chopped
capers
2 teaspoons finely chopped black
olives

½ teaspoon lemon juice
1 tablespoon minced parsley
2 cooked artichoke bottoms,
coated with lemon juice

Mix anchovies (optional), capers, olives, and lemon juice. Spoon into artichoke cavities. Completely cover with parsley. Chill.

If you have fresh leaves, arrange 12 in a fan shape around the stuffed artichoke placed at one side of each plate.

Note: The flavor of canned water-packed artichoke bottoms is improved by simmering them in homemade chicken stock before using. Fresh ones should be coated with lemon juice immediately after preparing to prevent discoloration.

CHICKEN CHASSEUR

(Each serving, 220 calories)

1 whole chicken breast, skinned
1 cup chicken broth
1 cup water
½ bay leaf
1 sprig fresh or ½ teaspoon dried thyme
⅓ stalk celery
½ teaspoon Golden Door seasoning salt (see page 277)
½ teaspoon olive oil

½ small onion, chopped
1 large clove garlic, minced
6 small mushrooms, sliced
2 small tomatoes, peeled and diced
oregano
¼ teaspoon dried or 1 tablespoon fresh tarragon
⅓ cup dry white wine
¼ teaspoon minced fresh chives
2 teaspoons minced fresh parsley

Cut breast in half and place in saucepan with chicken broth, water, bay leaf, thyme, celery, and salt. Cover and simmer for about 35 minutes, or until breast is tender. In the meantime, heat oil in a heavy skillet and add onion and garlic. Sauté until onion is limp. Add mushrooms and cook for 5 minutes. Add tomatoes, oregano, and tarragon and cook uncovered for about 20 minutes, stirring occasionally, until sauce thickens. Add wine and boil for 10 minutes.

Remove breast from cooking liquid; place each half in a serving dish or individual casserole with a little of the broth in the bottom. Just before serving add chives and parsley to the tomato wine sauce and spoon over chicken.

ZUCCHINI FORMAGGIO

(Each serving, 195 calories)

2 large zucchini, scrubbed but unpeeled
2 tablespoons 100% corn-oil margarine
salt

pepper
2 tablespoons grated Parmesan cheese
2 tablespoons minced parsley

Shave tips and stems off zucchini and grate on large holes of grater. Place zucchini in a colander set over a bowl. Let drain for 3 to 4 minutes. Just before cooking, squeeze gently by handfuls. (You may wish to reserve the vegetable juice you squeeze out to add to soups or stews.)

Melt margarine in a skillet. When bubbly, toss in the zucchini and add salt and pepper to taste. Cook until tender-crisp, about 3 to 5 minutes (taste to be sure). Add Parmesan cheese and parsley. Toss together and serve immediately.

QUICKIE

TURKEY SALAD DIVAN

(Each serving, 270 calories)

½ pound fresh broccoli
½ head butter lettuce

2 ounces Gruyère cheese, thinly sliced
¼ pound turkey, thinly sliced

Chive Dressing

½ cup plain low-fat yogurt
2 tablespoons minced chives
1 tablespoon minced parsley
2 teaspoons finely chopped green onion, including some of the green top

salt and pepper
pinch of dried crumbled tarragon
1 teaspoon Dijon mustard

In the morning, trim tough ends from the broccoli and split stalks through the flowerettes. Drop into boiling salted water to cover. Bring water back to a boil and cook, uncovered, for 3 to 5 minutes, or until stems can be easily pierced with a fork. Strain, rinse in cold water, and chill.

To make the dressing, mix together all dressing ingredients and chill.

In the evening, when ready to serve, arrange the lettuce, broccoli, cheese, and turkey on platter; pour dressing on top.

CARAMEL CUSTARD

(Each serving, 205 calories)

1 egg
⅔ cup nonfat milk
6 teaspoons sugar

grated peel of ½ lemon
100% corn-oil margarine

In a mixing bowl, beat egg and blend in milk, 3 teaspoons sugar, and lemon peel, stirring until the sugar dissolves.

Using margarine, grease 2 glass baking dishes or smoothly glazed custard cups of ½-cup size. Set in a baking pan containing 1 inch hot water.

Put 3 teaspoons sugar in heavy saucepan over low heat and stir until sugar melts and begins to brown. Quickly pour into prepared dishes. Cover with the custard mixture.

Bake at 325° F. for about 30 to 35 minutes, until centers no longer jiggle when pressed. Remove from water, cool, and chill.

To serve, loosen around top with knife and dip in hot water a little longer than you would to unmold gelatin. Hold plate over cup, invert quickly, and tap with knife handle or slap with palm to loosen.

BRUNCH OR LATE, LATE SUPPER

ZUCCHINI SALAD ANDALOUSE
(Each serving, 50 calories)

2 medium-sized zucchini	¼ teaspoon oregano
Golden Door seasoning salt	1 small red pimiento (fresh, if
(see page 277)	possible)
2 large shallots, finely chopped	dash of cayenne
1 clove garlic, finely chopped	1 medium-sized tomato
polyunsaturated oil	lettuce
1 tablespoon chopped chives	parsley
¼ teaspoon freshly ground	
black pepper	

Slice the zucchini into thin rounds, discarding the ends, and season lightly with seasoning salt and cayenne. In a heavy skillet sauté the shallots and garlic in a few drops of oil for a minute or two. Add the zucchini and cook quickly over high heat, stirring. Reduce the heat and cook, covered, for 3 to 4 minutes (zucchini should be slightly crisp). Transfer to a salad bowl and sprinkle with chives. Set aside to cool.

Peel the tomato and dice finely. Season with oregano. Mix well with the zucchini. Remove the core and seeds from the pimiento, dice, and add cayenne. Combine with the zucchini-tomato mixture.

Refrigerate the salad for 2 to 3 hours before serving on a bed of lettuce. Garnish with chopped fresh parsley.

PAUPIETTE OF VEAL ROULATINE
(Each serving, 400 calories)

2 veal scallopinis (about 3½ to 4 ounces each)
freshly ground black pepper
Golden Door seasoning salt (see page 277)
Italian seasoning
¾ pound fresh spinach
dash of nutmeg
½ cup grated Monterey Jack cheese
2 tablespoons freshly grated Parmesan cheese
2 tablespoons freshly toasted pine nuts
1 tablespoon 100% corn-oil margarine
⅛ cup dry white wine
juice of ½ small lemon
10 rigatoni noodles
¼ cup tomato juice
oregano
parsley

Pound the veal thin with the side of a cleaver (or ask the butcher to prepare it for you). Season each scallopini with seasoning salt, pepper, and Italian seasoning. Wash spinach and drain thoroughly. Cook in a tightly covered pan until slightly wilted. Drain thoroughly. Chop spinach coarsely and add seasoning salt, pepper, and nutmeg. In a saucepan combine spinach and Jack cheese. Cook over low heat until the cheese melts. Add the pine nuts and set aside to cool.

Spread each scallopini with half the spinach mixture and roll up, securing with toothpicks. In a heavy casserole brown the scallopini lightly in oil. Cover and bake in a 375° F. oven for 10 minutes. Remove from the oven and add the margarine and white wine. Squeeze the lemon juice over the top. Sprinkle the Parmesan over and return briefly to the oven or under the broiler.

Serve immediately—accompanied by the rigatoni noodles, which have been cooked until tender and then reheated in the tomato juice seasoned with oregano. Garnish the entire dish with parsley.

CREAM OF MANGO AU KIWI

(Each serving, 100 calories)

1 very ripe mango (fresh or canned)

½ cup fresh orange juice

1 tablespoon Grand Marnier

1 firm but ripe kiwi

Peel the mango, remove the stone, and put the pulp into the blender container. Add orange juice and blend for 2 to 3 minutes until creamy. In a small saucepan bring the liqueur to a boil (this removes approximately half the calories). Add the liqueur to the mango and blend again briefly. Divide the mango cream evenly between two dessert dishes. Peel the kiwi, slice into thin rounds, and arrange around the edge of the mango cream. Chill before serving.

DINNER FOR SIX

WHITE-WINE SPRITZER

(Each serving, 45 calories)

⅘ quart dry white wine (Chablis), well chilled

few dashes Angostura bitters

1 quart club soda or sparkling water, well chilled

lemon twists

Pour well-chilled wine into pitcher to half full. Add bitters and club soda. Serve immediately in large wineglasses or in highball glasses, with lemon twists.

Makes 12 servings (2 per person).

PEASANT CAVIAR

(Each serving, 85 calories with two crackers)

3 cups eggplant (about 1½ pounds)

2 tablespoons olive oil

1 teaspoon lemon juice

2 tablespoons minced onion

salt and pepper

6 black olives

parsley

12 rye wafers

The night before you plan to serve this appetizer, place the eggplant under the broiler on the lowest rack until the skin becomes charcoal black and eggplant is soft. Be sure to turn it occasionally. When done, peel off the skin without allowing eggplant to cool. Cube the pulp and whirl in the blender until creamy. Measure out 3 cups. Place in a bowl and add oil, lemon juice, onion, and salt and pepper to taste. Whip with a fork until fluffy. Refrigerate.

When ready to serve, garnish with olives and parsley and serve with rye wafers.

GOLDEN DOOR BREAST OF CHICKEN
(Each serving, 310 calories)

The chicken is stuffed with just a piece of cheese, which melts to look and taste like a rich sauce.

To bone chicken breasts: Bend breast halves until the large bone protrudes so you can pull it out. Use knife to loosen, if necessary. Then insert fingers under membrane with row of little bones; pull all off in one strip.

6 large boneless chicken-breast halves, skinned	1 tablespoon grated Parmesan or Romano cheese
6 strips Monterey Jack or Swiss cheese, each about 3 x 1 x 1/4 inches (about 1/4 pound)	salt and pepper
	3 tablespoons unbleached flour
	2 tablespoons salad or olive oil
3 eggs	parsley sprigs
1 tablespoon minced parsley	6 lemon wedges

Make a pocket for stuffing each chicken breast by slicing lengthwise from one side partially through. Lay cheese strip inside. Fasten opening with wooden pick; also fasten loose ends into a neat bundle (to be sure no opening remains where cheese may ooze out).

In a bowl, blend eggs, parsley, and grated cheese with salt and pepper to taste. Coat chicken heavily with flour, then roll it completely in the egg mixture.

Heat the oil in small frying pan over medium-high heat. Add chicken with as much egg clinging to it as possible. Spoon remaining egg mixture on top. Fry about 1 minute on each side, just enough to set the coating. (This much can be done ahead of serving time; then refrigerate.)

When ready to serve, place chicken in a baking pan and bake, uncovered, at 375° F. for 25 to 30 minutes, or until coating begins to brown. (If prepared ahead, let come to room temperature before cooking. A few extra minutes' baking may be required.) When you test chicken for doneness, be careful not to puncture where cheese may ooze out.

Remove picks and serve hot with parsley and lemon wedges.

GARDEN OF VEGETABLES

(Each serving, 110 calories)

2½ cups each raw cabbage, broccoli, cauliflower, and green beans (all cut according to instructions in recipe)

2 to 3 tablespoons water

3 tablespoons 100% corn-oil margarine

1 tablespoon salad oil or olive oil

4 cups spinach leaves, cut into 1-inch pieces

salt and pepper

Measure each after cutting: chop cabbage into ½-inch pieces; cut or break broccoli and cauliflower into ½-inch flowerettes; cut beans into ½-inch sections. Put water in saucepan, bring to a simmer, and immediately add all the vegetables *except* spinach. Dribble the oil over, cover, and simmer about 5 minutes—just until vegetables are tender-crisp. Drain in colander.

Put large frying pan or Chinese wok over highest heat, add margarine, and turn pan to coat. Add warm vegetables and spinach all at once. Stir and toss constantly for about 2 minutes while adding salt and pepper to taste, just until vegetables are very hot. Serve at once.

APPIAN PEARS

(Each serving, 175 calories)

3 large pears, peeled, halved, and cored

¾ cup sherry

6 tablespoons chopped slivered almonds

½ teaspoon almond extract

Put pears, cored sides up, in smallest possible baking dish. Dribble sherry over. Put almonds and almond extract into cavities. Bake uncovered at 350° F. for 30 minutes, basting with sherry occasionally. Serve hot or cold.

□ **WEEK II OF DINNER MENUS FOR WEIGHT REDUCTION**

		CALORIES
1 Very low cal	GAZPACHO	70
	CHILES RELLEÑOS RANCHO LA PUERTA	230
	TOSTADA SALAD	70
	TECATE SHERBET	125
	TOTAL:	495
2 Vegetarian	TOMATO AND CUCUMBER SALAD WITH MUSHROOMS	125
	GARDEN SPAGHETTI	400
	LEMON LIGHTNING	115
	TOTAL:	640
3 International	*SAKE* MARTINI	50
	CHICKEN LIVERS YAKITORI	150
	MIZUTAKI FOR TWO	315
	ORANGES IN SNOW	115
	TOTAL:	630
4 Golden Door Gourmet	CITY GARDEN SALAD	110
	FILLET OF SOLE IN EGG BATTER	100
	GREEN BEANS STUFATI	100
	CARROTS CREMATE	110
	FRUIT FOR DESSERT (OR FRUIT AND CHEESE)	210
	TOTAL:	630
5 Quickie	QUICK WELSH RAREBIT	330
	WALDORF SALAD	175
	TOTAL:	505

6	VEGETABLES BRAVADO	65
Brunch or late,	CHICKEN CACCIATORE	315
late supper	LETTUCE SALAD WITH CHEESE	
	DRESSING	135
	FRUIT FOR DESSERT (OR FRUIT AND	
	CHEESE)	100
	TOTAL:	615
7	SPARKLING SANGRIA	55
Dinner for six	OYSTERS IMPOSTOR	60
	TERIYAKI STEAK	300
	BAKED POTATOES ROMANOFF	130
	GOLDEN DOOR COMBINATION SALAD	165
	DESSERT À TAHITI	110
	TOTAL:	820

VERY LOW CAL

GAZPACHO

(Each serving, 70 calories)

1 small cucumber, peeled and seeded

3 medium-sized tomatoes, peeled

1 teaspoon red-wine vinegar

juice of 1 lemon

1 small clove garlic, cut up

dash of Worcestershire sauce

⅓ cup *each* diced green pepper, celery, and cucumber

Combine 1 cucumber, tomatoes, vinegar, lemon juice, garlic, and Worcestershire sauce in blender and blend until smooth. Refrigerate until ice cold. Serve topped with green pepper, celery, and cucumber.

CHILES RELLEÑOS RANCHO LA PUERTA

(Each serving, 230 calories)

1 teaspoon 100% corn-oil margarine

2 eggs, separated

⅛ teaspoon salt

1 tablespoon *each* unbleached flour and water, blended

1 (4-ounce) can diced green chiles (the mildly hot kind), drained

2 ounces (sliced about 1 x 2 x 3 inches) Monterey Jack or mild white Cheddar cheese (or ⅔ cup, shredded)

Chili powder

Grease with margarine a 9-inch pie pan or 2 casseroles of about 1½-cup capacity.

Beat egg whites with the salt until they hold soft peaks. Blend yolks with flour-water mixture until creamy. Gently fold whites into yolk mixture.

Spoon half the eggs into pan; distribute chiles on top, and then cheese. Cover completely with remaining egg mixture. With fingers, sprinkle enough chili powder on top to color delicately.

Bake at 325° F. for 20 to 25 minutes, or until puffy top is golden brown and feels firm. Serve at once.

TOSTADA SALAD
(Each serving, 70 calories)

½ head iceberg lettuce, cut into 4 wedges

A few garnishes typical of those used on a Mexican *tostada,* such as carrot curls, hot peppers, cucumber slices, radish roses, green pepper rings, or green onions

Guacamole Dressing (recipe follows)

paprika and cayenne

Arrange lettuce on 2 large plates and chill. Prepare garnishes and dressing. Pour dressing on lettuce and sprinkle with paprika and cayenne. Add garnishes at the side.

Guacamole Dressing
(Approximately 100 calories per recipe)

2 tablespoons lemon juice
1 tablespoon water
1 teaspoon honey
1 green onion

sliver of garlic
½ small, fully ripe avocado
salt and pepper

Combine ingredients in blender and blend, adding more water, if necessary, to make a creamy thick dressing. Season to taste.

TECATE SHERBET
(Each serving, 125 calories)

1 small, fully ripe papaya or large mango, peeled and seeded, or 2 medium-sized peaches, peeled

2 tablespoons *each* lemon juice and orange-flavored liqueur (or orange juice with a pinch of grated peel added)
2 orange slices

Cut fruit in chunks directly into blender container. Add lemon juice and liqueur. Purée, using a rubber spatula to scrape mixture down, and adding a little water if necessary.

Pour into 2 sherbet or champagne glasses and put in the freezer for 30 minutes to 1 hour. At serving time, slit each orange slice just to center and slip over glass edge.

Note: Dessert becomes too icy if frozen longer than 2 hours.

VEGETARIAN
TOMATO AND CUCUMBER SALAD WITH MUSHROOMS
(Each serving, 125 calories)

1 cup ricotta cheese
1 tablespoon corn oil or olive oil
1 tablespoon lime or lemon juice
salt and pepper
2 large ripe tomatoes, peeled and sliced

1 crisp medium-sized cucumber, peeled and sliced
4 mushrooms, thinly sliced
4 red radishes, thinly sliced
2 green onions, thinly sliced

To make the dressing, combine the ricotta cheese, oil, juice, and salt and pepper in the container of a blender and blend until smooth.

Place vegetables in bowl, pour dressing over vegetables, and toss lightly.

GARDEN SPAGHETTI
(Each serving, 400 calories)

The sauce is like a stew and you eat much more of it than of the starchy accompaniment.

¼ cup chopped onion
2 cloves garlic, minced
1 tablespoon olive oil
(approximate)
1½ cups unpeeled chopped
eggplant
½ cup chopped cauliflower
¼ cup chopped green pepper
2 large fresh mushrooms,
sliced
¼ cup minced fresh parsley
¼ teaspoon each thyme, crumbled bay leaf, and oregano

¼ teaspoon anise or fennel seed
(optional)
salt and pepper
1 (8-ounce) can tomato sauce
2 tablespoons red or white wine
(approximate)
4 ounces spaghetti or noodles
(green-spinach or whole-
wheat variety)
2 tablespoons grated Parmesan
cheese

In a large heavy pan, sauté onion and garlic in oil until limp. Add eggplant, cauliflower, green pepper, and mushrooms. Still until vegetables begin to brown; add an additional 1 teaspoon oil if they start to stick.

Add parsley, herbs, anise, salt, pepper, and tomato sauce. Stir until mixture boils; cover and lower heat. Simmer for 30 to 40 minutes, or until eggplant and cauliflower are no longer recognizable as such but are still in chunks (not puréed). Add wine shortly before cooking is finished (more, if necessary to thin sauce).

Cook spaghetti and drain. Arrange around rim of each large plate. Heap sauce in center and sprinkle on cheese.

LEMON LIGHTNING
(Each serving, 115 calories)

3 tablespoons ice-cold water
¼ cup nonfat dry-milk powder
3 tablespoons cold lemon juice
2 teaspoons sugar

¼ teaspoon vanilla extract
⅛ teaspoon almond extract
lemon (for grated peel)

Chill 2 sherbet dishes or custard cups. Put ice-cold water in mixing bowl and add milk. Beat with mixer until it resembles soft whipped cream. Dribble in lemon juice while beating. Sprinkle on sugar and flavoring while continuing to beat. Heap into dishes. Grate just a little peel on tops.

Eat at any stage—immediately, well-chilled, or frozen for about 1 to 1½ hours maximum (longer freezing produces ice crystals, but freezing just until firm gives rich sherbet texture).

INTERNATIONAL
SAKE MARTINI
(Each serving, 50 calories)

Many Japanese restaurants in America serve a martini made with rice wine, *sake,* which happens to be less caloric than gin or vodka.

¼ cup *sake*   1 strip lemon peel
1 or 2 teaspoons dry vermouth

Chill glasses. Shake wine with ice before pouring in. Add ice to glasses. Twist lemon to release oil into glass and drop in. Makes 1 serving.

CHICKEN LIVERS YAKITORI
(Each serving, 150 calories)

Yakitori, Japanese "shish kebab," may be made with chicken or beefsteak, as well as other ingredients such as mushrooms. Usually, *yakitori* is cooked over charcoal, but this recipe uses pan-broiling for greater ease and juiciness.

4 chicken livers, each cut into 3 pieces (if you are concerned over cholesterol, substitute parboiled skinless chicken breast)
3 green onions, white part only, cut into segments
½ green pepper, cut into 8 pieces
4 teaspoons soy sauce
2 teaspoons sugar

½ teaspoon grated fresh ginger root or ⅛ teaspoon ground ginger
1 teaspoon salad oil
salt
2 tablespoons water
Optional Japanese seasonings: *kona samsho* (ground pepper leaf) or *schichimi togarashi* (chili-sesame seasoning)

Use 4 thin metal or bamboo skewers, about 5 inches long (if they are bamboo, soak them in water so they will not burn.) Thread each with one-fourth of the livers, then onion, then pepper, and so on.

In a shallow plate, blend soy sauce, sugar, ginger, and several dashes salt. Marinate skewers in sauce for about 15 minutes, turning occasionally.

Heat oil in a frying pan or, using a pastry brush, coat a griddle large enough to hold skewers. Lay skewers in pan and cook 2 to 3 minutes, brushing with marinade; turn, and cook about 3 minutes more as you brush with marinade several times, using all of marinade. Dribble in the water and turn skewers in bubbly syrup just enough to glaze. Serve hot. Sprinkle with the Japanese seasonings, if available.

MIZUTAKI FOR TWO
(Each serving, 315 calories)

Mizutaki is a Japanese dish of chicken and vegetable pieces briefly cooked in water or broth and served with dipping sauce. Usually the cooking is ceremoniously done in special pots at the table. But you'll enjoy the dish more often if you don't make such a production number of it. This recipe lets you serve up steaming bowls of *mizutaki* in just a few minutes.

Substitute ingredients of similar caloric count when necessary.

4 cups chicken broth
(see page 278)
6 fresh mushrooms, sliced, or dried Oriental mushrooms (*shiitake*)
2 chicken-breast halves, skinned, boned, and cut into 12 pieces (for boning instructions, see Golden Door Breast of Chicken, page 226)
1 tablespoon soy sauce mixed with ½ teaspoon sugar
¼ cup sliced bamboo shoots
1 stalk celery, sliced diagonally into ½-inch chunks

1 carrot, sliced diagonally into ¼-inch pieces
1 (3-inch) piece Japanese white radish *(daikon)* or 1 small turnip, sliced into ¼-inch-thick rounds, each cut in half
½ green pepper, cut into 12 pieces of equal size
1 cup green vegetables (tightly packed Chinese cabbage, Chinese *bok choy,* or Swiss chard leaves cut or torn in large pieces)
4 green onions, sliced
Dipping Sauce (recipe follows)

Put broth into an 8-cup saucepan. If you use dried mushrooms, soak them in broth for about 15 minutes to soften, then cut out hard centers and cut each into 4 pieces.

Meanwhile, marinate chicken pieces in soy sauce-sugar mixture for at least 30 minutes, then drain.

Bring broth (with dried mushrooms, if used) to rolling boil; add chicken, bamboo shoots, celery, carrot, and radish. Simmer for 2 minutes. Add green pepper and fresh mushrooms, if used, and simmer for 1 more minute. Add green vegetable and green onion. Simmer about 1 more minute, or just until greens are slightly wilted.

Serve in large bowls with dipping sauce in dishes at the side. Remove foods from broth and dip in sauce. Finish by sipping broth.

Dipping Sauce

4 teaspoons toasted sesame seed	1 tablespoon sherry or Japanese
2 tablespoons soy sauce	sweet cooking wine (*mirin*)
2 teaspoons lemon or lime juice	1 thin slice fresh ginger root or
½ small clove garlic	⅛ teaspoon ground ginger
	1 teaspoon sugar

Pour all ingredients but 1 teaspoon sesame seed into blender and blend. Pour into sauce dishes and sprinkle with remaining sesame seed. (Sauce has about 100 calories.)

ORANGES IN SNOW

(Each serving, 115 calories)

In Japan a sweet similar to this, made with more sugar and agar-agar instead of gelatin, may be arranged in a black lacquer box as a gift. There the sweet is eaten at teatime. Sometimes fresh strawberry halves are used instead of mandarin oranges (or tangerines).

4 tangerines	1 egg white
1 teaspoon unflavored gelatin	⅛ teaspoon vanilla extract
1 tablespoon fresh lemon juice	1 drop almond extract
1 tablespoon sugar	

Squeeze 2 tangerines and add enough water to the juice to measure

⅓ cup. Combine in saucepan with gelatin, lemon juice, and sugar. Heat just to dissolve gelatin.

Beat egg white until it holds firm peaks. Still using rotary beater, very gradually pour in lukewarm gelatin mixture, vanilla extract, and almond extract, beating until well blended. Taste and add more flavorings if you like. Pour into 2 serving dishes. Chill while doing the following:

Peel and segment the remaining 2 tangerines. Remove all membrane and cut a tiny slit in each section to press out seeds. Lay tangerines in rows on top of "snow." Chill until firm.

GOLDEN DOOR GOURMET

CITY GARDEN SALAD

(Each serving, 110 calories)

Even in a city apartment, you can grow fresh salad greens at any time of the year—in a bottle. The greens are alfalfa sprouts, which are sweeter and milder than bean sprouts, not hay-like as the name sounds. You may be able to buy sprouts, but those you grow from seed sold in health-food stores are more alive with flavor and vitamins.

Following are instructions for growing alfalfa and a recipe for nippy dressing which enhances plain sprouts. Radishes may be a garnish. They have a complementary taste and look good chopped and mixed with your "crop."

Growing Alfalfa Sprouts: Put 1½ teaspoons seed in a wide-mouth quart (or larger) jar. Fill with slightly warm water. The next day, place a piece of fine screen wire or a fine wire strainer very tightly over jar and drain off water.

Dampen a towel and drape around jar to almost cover the opening. This keeps light out, lets air in, and prevents seeds from drying out.

Every morning and evening for 4 to 5 days, fill jar with room-temperature water, drain, and drape with damp towel. Sprouts are ready to eat when about 1 to 1½ inches long with little green leaves.

Remove seed hulls by putting sprouts into large bowl, filling with water repeatedly as you brush floating hulls off and drain sinking ones from bottom. A few hulls left in the bowl do not affect flavor, but too many are bitter. Drain sprouts. Eat right away or refrigerate in a bag with a paper towel.

Alfalfa Dressing
(185 calories per recipe)

1 tablespoon toasted sesame seed
1 tablespoon salad oil
2 tablespoons lemon juice
1 tablespoon water

1½ teaspoons Dijon mustard
¼ teaspoon paprika
1 teaspoon honey
freshly ground black pepper

Combine all ingredients in blender and blend.

FILLET OF SOLE IN EGG BATTER
(Each serving, 100 calories)

2 (3½-ounce) pieces fillet of sole or flounder
1 egg, well beaten

1 tablespoon minced fresh parsley
1 tablespoon minced fresh dill
1 teaspoon oil

Wash fish and drain. Combine egg with parsley and dill. Dip fish pieces lightly in egg on both sides (do not use all of egg). Heat oil in heavy skillet, and sauté fish until very lightly colored on bottom. Turn and sauté on other side. Remove fish to ovenproof plate covered with paper towel. Cover with aluminum foil and place in 400° F. oven for 2 to 3 minutes so that paper absorbs excess oil.

GREEN BEANS STUFATI
(Each serving, 100 calories)

½ pound fresh green beans
1 tablespoon 100% corn-oil margarine

Golden Door seasoning salt (see page 277) and pepper

String beans and snap each into 3 pieces. Steam for 7 to 9 minutes over boiling water. Drain in colander.

In large frying pan or Chinese wok, immediately melt margarine over high heat. When it sizzles, add the beans. Stir and toss constantly about 2 minutes while adding salt and pepper. Cook just until beans are slightly more tender and very hot. Serve at once.

CARROTS CREMATE
(Each serving, 110 calories)

Borrow this low-calorie creaming technique for use with other vegetables, meats, or seafood—even a quick curry of leftovers (about 1½ cups of whatever it may be).

4 medium-sized carrots, sliced	⅓ cup nonfat milk
2 teaspoons salad oil	salt and pepper
2 teaspoons unbleached flour	minced parsley

Cook carrots in smallest possible amount of boiling water just until tender-crisp. Drain well and continue preparation while still hot.

Put oil in small saucepan over medium-high heat; add carrots and toss until coated and hot. Sprinkle on flour and toss to coat. Remove from heat and stir in milk. Return to low heat and cook, stirring until sauce is smooth and thick (thin with water, if necessary). Add salt and pepper to taste. Garnish with parsley and serve immediately.

Curried Variation: For a hint of curry, sprinkle in ¼ teaspoon curry powder (or more) after adding carrots to oil. (For currying leftovers, sauté several tablespoons chopped onion in the oil before adding foods. Use additional curry powder to taste.)

FRUIT FOR DESSERT (OR FRUIT AND CHEESE)
(Each serving, 50 to 100 calories)

Complementary liqueurs can be sprinkled over fresh fruit for a simple and delicious dessert. Fresh fruit alone is also satisfying. Some examples:

1 cup fresh blueberries	90 calories
1 cup fresh strawberries	50 calories
1 peach	60 calories
1 pear	100 calories
1 cup diced pineapple	80 calories
1 orange	75 calories
1 apple	80 calories
½ cantaloupe	50 calories
4-inch wedge honeydew	60 calories

One ounce of any of the following cheeses adds about 110 calories: Cheddar, Edam, Gruyère, Monterey Jack, Port Salut, Muenster.

Try different combinations of fruit and cheese. Apple is the standard with Cheddar, but you may like other cheeses even better with apples.

QUICKIE

QUICK WELSH RAREBIT
(Each serving, 330 calories)

2 teaspoons arrowroot or cornstarch

½ teaspoon *each* dry mustard, paprika, and Worcestershire sauce

1 cup (4 ounces) shredded sharp natural Cheddar cheese

¼ cup cold water

3 slices whole-wheat bread (see Tecate Bread, page 279)

Mix arrowroot and seasonings with cheese in heavy saucepan or the top of a double boiler. Stir in water. Cook on low heat (or over boiling water), whisking or stirring constantly, until smooth and thick. (Makes ⅓ cup sauce.)

Toast bread. Cut each slice crosswise to form 4 triangles. Arrange 4 triangles around edge of each plate, spoon half the sauce inside and lay 2 triangles on sauce.

Broiled Sandwich Variation: Cool sauce until the consistency of a spread. Toast bread. Spread cheese to edges and broil until bubbly.

WALDORF SALAD
(Each serving, 175 calories)

2 small unpeeled red apples, cored and diced

an equal amount of diced celery

2 tablespoons mayonnaise (see page 276)

lettuce leaves

2 tablespoons coarsely chopped walnuts

Toss apples and celery with the mayonanise. Heap on lettuce-lined plates. Sprinkle walnuts on top.

VEGETABLES BRAVADO
(Each serving, 50 to 65 calories)

cracked ice
1 small celery heart or small head
    fresh fennel
1 carrot, cut in sticks or curls

6 cherry tomatoes
2 sprigs parsley or watercress
Blue-cheese dip (recipe follows)

Fill 2 very large goblets or brandy snifters (or a bowl) with ice. Cut celery or fennel into thick slices, straight through root end, and trim tops attractively. Press upright into ice. Add carrot and tomatoes. Garnish with parsley. Serve with dip. Eat as an appetizer.

Blue-Cheese Dip
(Approximately 150 calories in recipe)

¼ cup plain, skim-milk yogurt
1½ teaspoons blue cheese or
    Roquefort

½ cup pot cheese

Combine ingredients and mix well. Chill. Use ¼ cup per person.

CHICKEN CACCIATORE
(Each serving, 315 calories)

2 chicken-breast halves, skinned
    and boned (for boning instruc-
    tions, see Golden Door Breast
    of Chicken, page 226)
2 teaspoons salad oil or olive oil
¼ cup chopped onion
1 small clove garlic, minced
¾ cup chopped fresh or canned
    tomatoes (preferably Italian
    plum type) plus extra juice
    as needed

salt and freshly ground black
    pepper
¼ teaspoon each crumbled bay
    leaf, thyme, and marjoram
¼ cup dry white wine
½ small green pepper, cut into
    12 pieces
6 fresh mushrooms
    (about 4 ounces), sliced
1 tablespoon 100% corn-oil
    margarine

Cut chicken breast into 12 pieces. In deep frying pan or pot with lid, heat 1 teaspoon oil over high heat. Sauté chicken until lightly browned and remove with a slotted spoon. Add remaining 1 teaspoon oil, onion, and garlic. Sauté until golden. Add tomatoes, salt, pepper, and herbs. Cover and simmer for 15 minutes.

Add chicken and wine; cover and simmer for 5 minutes. Add green pepper; cover and simmer for 10 minutes. Add mushrooms and margarine. Increase heat and cook rapidly, uncovered, stirring often, until mushrooms are soft and sauce looks creamy.

LETTUCE SALAD WITH CHEESE DRESSING
(Each serving, 135 calories)

4 cups lettuce (several varieties)
3 tablespoons low-fat buttermilk
2 teaspoons corn or olive oil
1 teaspoon red- or white-wine vinegar

1 ounce blue cheese (or a mild cheese such as Monterey Jack, crumbled)
1 drop Worcestershire sauce
coarsely ground black pepper

Tear lettuce into bite-sized pieces and arrange on salad plates.

In blender, combine all remaining ingredients except pepper. Blend and pour over lettuce. Sprinkle pepper on liberally.

DINNER FOR SIX
SPARKLING SANGRIA
(Each serving, 55 calories)

For each serving
¼ cup each red wine and club soda (sparkling water)

1 tablespoon fresh orange juice
¼ thin slice each orange and lemon

Combine in tumbler or wineglass with ice cubes.
For 12 servings

Combine ⅘ quart red wine, ¾ quart club soda, ¾ cup orange juice, and 3 slices each orange and lemon, quartered.

OYSTERS IMPOSTOR
(Each serving, 60 calories)

This appetizer (which can also be a main dish) is a poor-in-calories country cousin masquerading as the much richer Oysters Rockefeller.

1 pound fresh spinach
12 raw oysters (preferably blue-
    points), each scrubbed and
    opened, on a half-shell
hot-pepper sauce

1 cup shredded Monterey Jack
    cheese
paprika
6 lemon wedges

Cook spinach slowly in its own moisture in a tightly covered pan until just slightly tender but still brilliant green. Drain, chop, and press out as much liquid as possible.

Arrange oysters in shell on baking pan. Shake 2 drops hot-pepper sauce on each. Cover each with spinach (about 1 heaping tablespoon). Sprinkle cheese on top. Sprinkle liberally with paprika.

Bake at 375° F. for about 10 minutes, or until the oysters underneath are very hot. Serve at once with lemon wedges.

TERIYAKI STEAK

(Each serving, 300 calories)

This recipe is for pan-broiling, which most chefs prefer because the meat stays juicier and a sauce is made naturally. However, the marinated meat also can be oven or charcoal broiled.

6 (4-ounce) boneless steaks, such
    as New York strip or sirloin,
    ½-inch thick and trimmed of
    all fat
¼ cup soy sauce
12 paper-thin slices fresh ginger

root or ½ teaspoon ground
    ginger
1 large clove garlic, crushed
2 tablespoons dark brown sugar
1 tablespoon polyunsaturated
    oil
2 tablespoons water

Place all ingredients except oil and water in bowl. Turn meat in marinade at least 10 minutes, or until it warms up to room temperature.

Brush the oil over a cold frying pan. Drain steaks, pat dry with paper towel, and lay in pan. Turn heat on medium high and cook 4 minutes on each side for medium rare. Ginger slices may be browned to use as garnish.

Remove meat and keep warm on heated plates. Turn off heat. Pour the water into the pan and stir to deglaze pan. Spoon sauce, as much as you like, over steaks. Top with ginger slices.

BAKED POTATOES ROMANOFF

(Each serving, 130 calories)

6 small baking potatoes
½ cup each low-fat yogurt and low-fat cottage cheese

salt and pepper
1 (1-ounce) jar black caviar (lumpfish type is fine)

Bake potatoes at 375° F. until tender. Meanwhile, mix yogurt and cheese in blender until thickened like sour cream.

Slit each potato down the middle lengthwise and twice crosswise. Press from both sides to puff potato upward and spread open. Season with salt and pepper. Spoon on yogurt-cheese. Top each potato with a dab of caviar.

GOLDEN DOOR COMBINATION SALAD

(Each serving, 165 calories)

3 cups torn lettuce, preferably a mixture of several kinds
½ cup each raw cauliflowerettes, broccoli flowerettes, raw bean sprouts, and slivered green or red pepper

6 tablespoons corn or olive oil
¼ cup fresh lemon juice
1 teaspoon Dijon mustard
1 clove garlic, crushed
salt and pepper
2 fully ripe tomatoes, chopped

Put lettuce and vegetables in large mixing bowl. Blend all remaining ingredients *except* tomato for dressing. Serve in individual salad bowls. Top each with a spoonful of tomato.

DESSERT À TAHITI

(Each serving, 110 calories)

2 cups chopped fresh pineapple
3 eggs
1 cup nonfat milk
2 tablespoons sugar

1 teaspoon vanilla extract
1½ teaspoons orange-flavored liqueur
orange (for grated peel)

In the top of a double boiler, combine eggs, milk, and sugar; whisk to blend egg thoroughly. Cook over boiling water. When mixture begins to thicken, stir continuously until the consistency of heavy cream—the custard will not get very thick. Remove from heat and blend in liqueur and vanilla extract. Cool to room temperature.

Pour custard over pineapple. Grate a little orange peel for a garnish. Chill before serving (either in the pineapple shell or in 2 champagne or sherbet glasses).

□ WEEK III OF DINNER MENUS FOR WEIGHT REDUCTION

		CALORIES
1 Very low cal	SPINACH SOUP	170
	MEAT-PATTY PLATTER	335
	ZIGZAG MELON ESCONDIDO	40
	TOTAL:	545
2 Vegetarian	COLD CUCUMBER SOUP	90
	MARINATED VEGETABLE MAZA	70
	TABBOULEH SALAD	280
	CHEESE WEDGE	110
	TOTAL:	550
3 International	OYSTERS AT SEA	45
	LILY POND WAN	35
	FISH SHIOYAKI	300
	CUCUMBER-CELERY SUNOMO	40
	FRUIT FOR DESSERT	100
	TOTAL:	520
4 Golden Door Gourmet	MEDITERRANEAN TOMATO SALAD	65
	CHICKEN PAPRIKASH	270
	EGGPLANT HUNGARIAN	105
	SLIM PEACH MELBA	85
	TOTAL:	525

5	GUACAMOLE-STUFFED MUSHROOMS	110
Quickie	POT-AU-FEU	430
	TIPSY PINEAPPLE HAWAIIAN	115
	TOTAL:	655

6	FRESH GREEN BEAN SALAD	130
Brunch or late,	SHRIMP-STUFFED FISH	265
late supper	COEUR À LA CRÈME	175
	TOTAL:	570

7	FRUIT-FROSTED WINE	55
Dinner for six	CAVIAR MOUSSE	75
	FOIL-BAKED CHICKEN	175
	BAKED STUFFED TOMATO	200
	RAW MUSHROOM SALAD	145
	BANANA ICE CREAM	100
	TOTAL:	750

VERY LOW CAL

SPINACH SOUP

(Each serving, 170 calories)

1 pound fresh spinach
1 tablespoon 100% corn-oil
  margarine
¼ cup finely chopped onion
1 clove garlic, minced
1 teaspoon whole-wheat flour

2 cups chicken broth
  (see recipe page 278)
salt and pepper
2 tablespoons grated Parmesan
  cheese

Wash spinach carefully to remove any grit or sand, and chop.

In a heavy skillet, melt the margarine and sauté the onion and garlic until golden. Add the spinach. Cover tightly and steam over low heat for about 3 minutes, or until spinach is wilted. Stir in the flour and add chicken broth. Simmer for 5 minutes. Season to taste with salt and pepper.

Purée the soup in a blender; reheat to serve, and sprinkle with Parmesan cheese.

MEAT-PATTY PLATTER

(Each serving, 335 calories)

½ pound ground round steak
   (without fat)
2 lettuce leaves
1 large tomato cut into 4 slices
watercress sprigs

2 thin slices Monterey Jack or
   Swiss cheese
catsup and/or mayonnaise
   (see pages 274 and 276)

Form beef into 2 oblong patties. Pat firmly with the flat side of a wide knife blade and then score gently in a crisscross pattern on both sides while rounding edges a bit. (This makes meat look attractive and also keeps it from cracking as it cooks.)

For each serving, arrange on a dinner plate a lettuce leaf topped with 2 tomato slices and a bed of watercress.

Cook patties in a heated frying pan for 2 minutes; turn and cover. Cook until hot, uncover, and lay cheese on top. Cover again and cook about 2 minutes more, until patty has browned on bottom and cheese melts a little. Lay meat beside watercress and decorate with a dollop of catsup and/or mayonnaise.

ZIGZAG MELON ESCONDIDO

(Each serving, 40 calories)

2 lengthwise wedges cantaloupe,
   honeydew, or Persian melon
2 sprigs fresh mint (optional)

2 large strawberries
2 lemon wedges

Zigzag each wedge: First, at each tip make crosswise cut just to the rind. Then slice inward from the cut close to rind all the way underneath to reach the other end, and free melon in one piece.

Put melon, still on rind, on a plate. Cut crosswise into 6 pieces of equal width. Pull the first about ½ inch to one side, the next ½ inch to the other side, and so on to zigzag all pieces. Lay mint, berry, and lemon in a row at the center of each melon.

Pineapple Variation: Fresh pineapple can also be prepared this way.

VEGETARIAN
COLD CUCUMBER SOUP
(Each serving, 90 calories)

This quick blender combination makes a soup you can sip like a cocktail before dinner.

1 cup low-fat yogurt
½ cup water
½ small clove garlic
8 fresh mint leaves or
¼ teaspoon dried crumbled mint
⅛ teaspoon dried dill weed or several sprigs fresh dill
1 cucumber
salt

Put yogurt, water, garlic, and herbs in blender. Cut a small slice of unpeeled cucumber off either end and reserve for garnish. Peel rest of cucumber, cut in half, scoop out and discard seeds. Cut in small pieces into blender container. Blend until creamy. Add salt to taste.

Serve in cocktail or champagne glasses. Cut a slit to the center of each reserved cucumber slice and slip over glass rim. Chill thoroughly. Serve with a floating ice cube.

MARINATED VEGETABLE MAZA
(Each serving, 70 calories)

Throughout the Near and Middle East, *maza* or *meze* means appetizer.

2 raw turnips, thinly sliced
2 carrots, scraped and thinly sliced
½ cup pickled-beet juice or the following blend: ½ cup juice
drained from cooked beets, mixed with 1 tablespoon vinegar, 1 teaspoon sugar, and a sprinkling of salt

Marinate vegetables in beet juice for at least 15 minutes or for several hours, turning to make sure turnips become deep pink and carrots deep red-orange. Drain before serving.

TABBOULEH SALAD

(Each serving, 280 calories)

This Arabic salad has universal appeal. With a little effort you can find bulgur almost anywhere now. Bulgur comes in three forms—large almost-whole grains (the type also to use for pilaf), medium-sized cracked, and very finely cracked. The medium size is the best for *tabbouleh*, but the more frequently found large size works fine.

½ cup bulgur
2 large, fully ripe tomatoes, finely chopped
1 small green bell pepper, finely chopped
1 small cucumber, peeled and finely chopped
6 small green onions, including part of tops, finely chopped
6 radishes, finely chopped
1 cup finely minced parsley (about 2 large bunches)

1 tablespoon minced fresh-mint leaves
Dressing (recipe follows)
lemon wedges for garnish, and lettuce leaves
nutmeg (optional)
Optional garnishes: tomato wedges, green-pepper rings, cucumber slices, small green onions, radish roses, parsley, or mint leaves

Cover bulgur with water by at least 1 inch and soak until soft but still slightly crunchy—about 30 minutes. Strain and press out excess water.

Combine with chopped vegetables, parsley, and mint. Dribble dressing over and toss with fork. Let salad marinate for about 15 minutes, or chill as long as several hours. Make beds of lettuce leaves on large plates, heap salad in centers, add lemon wedges and optional garnishes. Pass nutmeg to sprinkle on salad, if desired.

Dressing

2 tablespoons olive oil
2 tablespoons fresh lemon juice
½ teaspoon salt
½ teaspoon allspice (optional)
½ teaspoon dry mustard

¼ teaspoon freshly ground black pepper
Dash of hot-pepper sauce or cayenne
1 small clove garlic, pressed

Combine ingredients and mix well. Pour over salad.

INTERNATIONAL
OYSTERS AT SEA
(Each serving, 45 calories)

For serving you will need 2 plates or bowls, preferably pottery or straw; pebbles, similar to those sold for flower arrangements; and 2 tiny sauce cups or extra oyster shells.

6 raw oysters, on the half-shell
1 tablespoon each Japanese rice-wine vinegar (or regular distilled white vinegar) and fresh lemon juice
½ teaspoon soy sauce

1 teaspoon grated Japanese white radish (*daikon*) or regular red radish or turnip
¼ teaspoon grated fresh ginger root

Line plates with pebbles. On each plate arrange 3 oysters on half-shells, with a sauce cup. Blend vinegar and lemon juice, and sprinkle oysters with one-fourth of mixture. For dipping sauce, blend the remaining vinegar-lemon mixture with soy sauce, radish, and ginger. Pour into sauce dishes.

LILY POND WAN
(Each serving, 35 calories)

Wan is very clear soup containing tidbits of colorful vegetables that create a still life when presented in a simple classic soup bowl of black or Chinese-red lacquer.

2 cups clear chicken broth (see recipe page 278) or Japanese *dashi* broth (instructions follow)
2 paper-thin slices carrot

2 very small spinach leaves or watercress sprigs
1 paper-thin slice lemon, cut in half

Heat broth, add carrot, and simmer for 1 minute, or just until carrot turns bright orange. Pour broth into Japanese bowls and put a carrot slice in each. Slip leaf and lemon into each "pond." Serve hot. Sip from the bowl.

Instructions for Dashi Broth: Buy a box of ingredients labeled *dashi-no-moto* soup stock (it comes in either pellet form or in little bags resembling tea bags). Many supermarkets carry this in the gourmet or Oriental section. Brew according to package directions. For clear broth, do not press bag; remove gently. Let broth cool and settle. Pour off clear top for Lily Pond Wan. Refrigerate or freeze remainder. *Dashi* is the broth you should use for sukiyaki or tempura dipping sauce.

FISH SHIOYAKI

(Each serving, 300 calories)

The Japanese method of *shio* (salt) *yaki* (broiling) produces the most delicious fish. For genuine *shioyaki* the fish must have skin on it. Salt is sprinkled on skin only, never on the flesh. That is why the large amount of salt does not make the fish taste salty.

2 small whole fish (about ⅓ pound each) or 1 larger fish weighing ⅔ pound	cabbage (lettuce for delicate fish, cabbage for stronger-flavored types)
salt	1 thick slice each orange and
⅔ cup finely shredded lettuce or	lemon, both cut in half

Fresh- or saltwater fish may be used. A good choice is rainbow trout or a sea fish of similar size and shape. Small whole fish with head and tail intact cook more easily and look best. But fish without head or tail, or pieces with skin on can be used. Fish must be fully cleaned internally, and scaled.

Fish should be at room temperature and patted dry with paper towel before cooking. Oil head and tail to prevent drying.

To cook, line broiler pan with foil. Preheat broiler with rack about 6 inches below. (Fish could also be charcoal-broiled.)

Cut about 3 diagonal slashes at intervals on each side of fish, just through skin. Lay fish on pan and sprinkle *heavily* with salt. (If you like to eat fish skin, use about twice as much salt as you would use for meat. If you don't eat the skin, salt even more heavily.) *Do not* salt inside fish or on flesh anywhere.

Broil about 3 to 4 minutes for ⅓-pound fish or 5 minutes for ⅔-pound fish. Turn, again salt heavily, cover tail with foil to prevent burning; broil about the same amount of time again. Skin of fish will be blistered and crispy; salt will be partially white and somewhat browned.

Meanwhile, prepare serving plates with a row of shredded vegetable down one side of each. Lay fish beside vegetable; place orange half between, and lemon half atop orange. Serve both fish and salad completely plain, or with a few drops of citrus juice from the garnish.

CUCUMBER-CELERY SUNOMO

(Each serving, 40 calories)

Sunomo is the Japanese word for dishes resembling salads.

1 cucumber
2 stalks celery
3 tablespoons Japanese rice-wine vinegar or regular distilled white vinegar
1 tablespoon water

2 teaspoons sugar
2 teaspoons *sake* (Japanese rice wine) or dry sherry (optional)
¼ teaspoon salt
¼ teaspoon grated fresh ginger root (optional)

Prepare the garnishes first: Cut 2 "ribbons" of cucumber peel about 6 inches long and ½ inch wide. Trim edges evenly. Tie each in a single, loose knot. Also reserve 2 tiny celery-leaf clusters.

Finish peeling cucumber; cut in half lengthwise; scoop out seeds and discard them. Slice paper-thin. Slice celery diagonally paper-thin. Toss together in bowl.

Blend remaining ingredients and pour over salad. Toss, taste, and add salt, if necessary. Chill.

Heap into two small bowls. Perch cucumber knot on each mound and tuck celery leaves inside knot.

GOLDEN DOOR GOURMET

MEDITERRANEAN TOMATO SALAD

(Each serving, 65 calories)

2 large romaine leaves
1 large, fully ripe tomato, cut into 4 slices
salt and pepper
fresh parsley

2 lemon wedges
1 teaspoon fresh or ¼ teaspoon dried oregano
2 teaspoons olive oil

For each serving: Lay leaf on plate, top with 2 tomato slices, and season with salt and pepper. Tuck parsley sprig at side and garnish with 1 lemon wedge.

Mince ½ teaspoon parsley and mix with oregano. Sprinkle on tomatoes, then dribble oil on. Squeeze lemon on for tartness as desired.

CHICKEN PAPRIKASH

(Each serving, 270 calories)

Paprika is the most typical Hungarian seasoning. Hungarian cooks use it to flavor and thicken sauces, as well as for color. Ground from dried capsicum peppers, paprika comes in a wide spectrum of pungency, from very hot to sweetly mild.

1 pound frying-chicken pieces (white meat)	1 sliver garlic, minced pinch of pepper
½ cup water	½ cup plain low-fat yogurt
¼ pound fresh mushrooms, sliced	1 tablespoon sweet Hungarian paprika
½ onion, sliced	
½ cup chopped green pepper	

Place chicken pieces, skin side down, in a skillet. Add 2 tablespoons water. Cover and cook very slowly over medium heat until the water evaporates and the chicken begins to brown in its own fat. Add mushrooms, onion, green pepper, and garlic and brown slowly. Pour off fat that has accumulated in the pan.

Add the remaining water. Cover and simmer for 35 to 40 minutes or until chicken is tender. Remove chicken from pan and keep warm.

Skim any fat from the surface of the pan juices. Stir in yogurt and paprika and cook over low heat until warmed through. *Do not boil.*

Pour sauce over chicken and serve immediately.

EGGPLANT HUNGARIAN

(Each serving, 105 calories)

1 small eggplant (preferably long Italian style)	oregano
Golden Door seasoning salt (see page 277)	2 teaspoons polyunsaturated oil parsley

Wash the eggplant, remove the ends, and slice lengthwise. Make shallow crosswise incisions with a knife. Sprinkle with seasonings and a teaspoon of polyunsaturated oil. Bake in a 350° F. oven for 30 to 40 minutes. Serve immediately.

SLIM PEACH MELBA
(Each serving, 85 calories)

2 fresh peaches, peeled and halved
¼ cup low-fat yogurt
2 teaspoons honey

several dashes of nutmeg
¼ cup chopped fresh strawberries or raspberries
lime (for grated peel)

Arrange 1 peach half in each of 2 sherbet or champagne glasses.

Into blender put yogurt, 1 teaspoon honey, nutmeg, and 1 peach half, cut in small pieces. Purée. Chop last peach half and add to sauce (do not blend). Pour into glasses.

Blend berries with remaining 1 teaspoon honey and spoon into peach centers. Grate on lime peel.

QUICKIE
GUACAMOLE-STUFFED MUSHROOMS
(Each serving, 110 calories)

¼ pound medium-sized mushrooms
1½ teaspoons lemon juice
½ teaspoon salt

½ ripe avocado
1 teaspoon finely minced onion
dash of hot-pepper sauce
1 tablespoon diced tomato

Wipe mushrooms clean. Remove stems and reserve for other uses. Brush insides of caps with half the lemon juice and sprinkle with a bit of salt. Mash avocado and blend in remaining lemon juice, salt, onion, and hot-pepper sauce. Mix well. Fill each cap with a tablespoon of the mixture and garnish with some diced tomato.

POT-AU-FEU
(Each serving, 430 calories)

This dish must be prepared the day before it is to be served. After it is refrigerated overnight, the fat, which has risen to the top, is easy to remove. The dish improves in flavor by sitting for 12 to 24 hours.

For two servings, only ½ the meat is served. The remaining meat is excellent in a cold salad. Any leftover broth can be frozen and used as a soup base.

1 pound beef rump or round (lean only), cut into cubes	1½ cups mixed coarsely chopped vegetables (onion, carrots, celery, white turnips, parsnips—whatever suits your taste)
1 teaspoon salt	
1 *bouquet garni* (1 bay leaf, ¼ teaspoon thyme, ½ teaspoon peppercorns, 1 clove garlic, 3 whole cloves, 4 sprigs parsley, and a few celery leaves tied in a cheesecloth bag or placed in a tea ball)	2 leeks, white part only, sliced
	2 carrots, peeled and quartered
	2 potatoes, washed

Place the meat in a heavy soup kettle with water to cover. Add the salt and *bouquet garni*. Bring to a boil, skimming the foam from the top as it rises. Reduce the heat and simmer, covered, until the meat is almost tender, about 3 hours. Discard the *bouquet garni* and correct the seasoning. Refrigerate.

When ready to serve, remove the accumulated fat from the top and reheat. Add the vegetables, except the potatoes, and simmer until tender, about 30 minutes. Meanwhile cook the potatoes separately, until tender. Peel, quarter, and add to pot-au-feu. Serve half of the meat.

Some people prefer their pot-au-feu served with the meat in the broth, but the French prefer to sip the broth first and then eat the meat. Serve with *cornichons* (small European sour pickles) and Dijon mustard or horseradish sauce.

TIPSY PINEAPPLE HAWAIIAN
(Each serving, 115 calories)

½ small fresh pineapple	2 tablespoons shredded coconut, plain or toasted
2 teaspoons rum or orange-flavored liqueur (optional)	

Cut pineapple in half lengthwise right through leaves and reserve half for other uses. Cut other half in two lengthwise, again right through leaves. With a small knife, cut out cores. Cut between rind and fruit to loosen completely, but leave in place. Cut fruit in chunks by slicing each serving lengthwise through the middle and crosswise five or six times.

Sprinkle liqueur along centers. Top with coconut.

BRUNCH OR LATE, LATE SUPPER
FRESH GREEN BEAN SALAD
(Each serving, 130 calories)

¾ pound green beans (young, tender, and fresh)
1 teaspoon finely chopped shallots
1 teaspoon chopped fresh parsley

1 to 2 tablespoons vinaigrette dressing (see Golden Door Combination Salad, page 243)
lettuce
pimiento strips

Cut the ends from the beans; remove strings and slice beans lengthwise. Blanch in boiling salted water for 2 to 3 minutes. Drain and cool immediately (the beans must still be green and crisp). Add the shallots and parsley. When ready to serve, blend in the dressing. Serve the salad on a bed of lettuce with additional parsley sprinkled on top. Decorate each portion with crossed strips of red pimiento.

SHRIMP-STUFFED FISH
(Each serving, 265 calories)

2 (⅓-pound) fish fillets, such as flounder or sole
½ cup (about 2 ounces) tiny shrimp or larger shrimp, cut up
2 fresh mushrooms, halved and sliced
5 saltines, crushed
3 tablespoons nonfat dry-milk powder

1 egg
2 teaspoons lemon juice
salt and pepper
2 teaspoons polyunsaturated oil
1 tablespoon minced parsley
1 tablespoon dry white wine or dry vermouth

Lay each fillet flat. With small sharp-pointed knife, cut a slit length-wise down the center, about halfway through only. Make pockets for stuffing on both sides of slit by cutting from within slit nearly through to each edge. (The fillet, slit with pockets on each side, should resemble wrapping used for individual packets of facial tissue.)

Combine shrimp, mushrooms, crackers, milk powder, egg, lemon juice, and salt and pepper to taste. Blend with a fork.

Oil 2 individual oblong ramekins or 2 pieces of aluminum foil. Lay fish in (bring foil up around sides to make a sort of boat) and lay on baking pan. Stuff fish with shrimp mixture. Tuck ends of fish under; brush sides with 2 teaspoons oil, sprinkle parsley over stuffing, and pour wine into container.

Bake uncovered at 375° F. for 10 to 15 minutes, or until fish flakes easily when tested with fork.

COEUR À LA CRÈME
(Each serving, 175 calories)

This is a low-calorie version of the classic French dessert.

½ cup low-fat creamed cottage cheese

½ (3-ounce) package Neufchatel cheese, slightly softened

pinch of salt

2 tablespoons sugar

¾ cup fresh strawberries

In the morning, thoroughly blend cheeses, salt, and sugar in a bowl. Refrigerate.

About 15 minutes before serving, form the cheese into a heart shape, place on a platter, and surround with berries.

DINNER FOR SIX
FRUIT-FROSTED WINE
(Each serving, 55 calories)

⅘ quart dry white wine, like Chablis, chilled

1 quart club soda, chilled

1 large peach, cut in 12 slices

12 large strawberries

Just before serving, combine ingredients in large glass pitcher. Serve over ice. Makes 12 servings (two glasses per person).

CAVIAR MOUSSE

(Each ¼ cup, 55 calories; 20 calories per 2 crackers)

1 envelope (1 tablespoon)
  unflavored gelatin
2 tablespoons cold water
½ cup boiling water
1 tablespoon lemon juice
2 tablespoons mayonnaise (see
  page 276)

dash of hot-pepper sauce
2 teaspoons minced shallots
4 ounces (½ cup) red caviar or
  chopped olives
2 cups plain low-fat yogurt
watercress
melba toast or rye thins

Soften gelatin in cold water. Add boiling water and stir until dissolved. Cool slightly, then stir in lemon juice, mayonnaise, hot-pepper sauce, shallots, caviar, and yogurt. Rinse 3½- to 4-cup mold with cold water; drain, and spoon in caviar mixture. Chill until set (2 to 3 hours). Unmold and serve on a bed of watercress, accompanied by crackers.

FOIL-BAKED CHICKEN

(Each serving, 175 calories)

6 small whole chicken breasts or
  6 large halves, skinned and
  boned
salt
6 tablespoons minced celery

6 tablespoons minced onion
2 tablespoons minced fresh parsley
6 tablespoons lemon juice
6 tablespoons dry white wine or
  dry vermouth

Cut six squares (18 x 18 inches) of aluminum foil. Place a breast on each square and sprinkle with salt, celery, onion, and parsley. Add lemon juice and wine to each package. Pull four corners of foil up to make a tight bundle around chicken. Place packages in shallow baking pan and bake at 375° F. for 35 minutes. Serve hot, or chilled with juice jelled around chicken.

BAKED STUFFED TOMATO

(Each serving, 200 calories)

6 large tomatoes
1½ cups diced Monterey Jack
  cheese
¾ cup dry bread crumbs

¾ teaspoon tarragon
¾ teaspoon sweet basil
pepper and salt
  3 cloves garlic, pressed

Cut tops off tomatoes and scoop out centers. Seed and chop the pulp. Lightly sprinkle the inside of each scooped-out tomato with salt. Mix tomato pulp with remaining ingredients, and spoon into the tomatoes. Bake at 375° F. for 15 minutes, or until bubbly.

RAW MUSHROOM SALAD
(Each serving, 145 calories)

36 fresh mushrooms, thinly sliced
2 tablespoons lemon juice
2 tablespoons wine vinegar
4 tablespoons polyunsaturated oil
2 tablespoons chopped green onion
2 tablespoons minced chives
2 tablespoons minced fresh parsley
Golden Door seasoning salt (see page 277)
freshly ground black pepper
lettuce leaves
alfalfa sprouts (see page 236)

Place mushrooms in a bowl. Toss with lemon juice and vinegar. Add oil, green onion, chives, parsley, seasoning salt, and pepper. Toss again. Chill before serving.

When ready to serve, select a few handsome leaves of lettuce and place on two individual salad plates. Cover with a small mound of alfalfa sprouts and the marinated mushrooms.

BANANA ICE CREAM
(Each serving, 100 calories)

6 small bananas (fully ripe but not overripe)
lemon juice
1½ teaspoons vanilla extract
¾ cup cold nonfat milk or water (approximate)

Peel bananas; cut out any brown spots and cut off tips. Carefully remove all tiny strings down the sides or any imperfection (black spot or bruise). Squeeze lemon juice all over to prevent discoloration. Wrap each banana tightly in plastic wrap. Freeze solid. Chill 2 sherbet or champagne glasses.

At serving time, put vanilla and milk into the blender container. Quickly cut bananas into small chunks directly into container. Blend;

turn blender on and off and scrape mixture down with a rubber spatula, as necessary, until smooth and creamy. Add more cold milk if ice cream gets too thick to blend fully. Pour into chilled glasses. (Dessert may be held in freezer a few minutes before serving, but do not refreeze—ice crystals form.)

Banana-Strawberry Variation: Combine 1 frozen banana with about 6 large frozen strawberries.

□ WEEK IV OF DINNER MENUS FOR WEIGHT REDUCTION

		CALORIES
1 Very low cal	BROILED SHRIMP	210
	GREEN SALAD WITH ONION AND ORANGE	90
	PALACE MUHALLEBI	130
	TOTAL:	430
2 Vegetarian	WATER CHESTNUTS RUMAKI	75
	FRESH FRUIT PLATE WITH PEACH DRESSING	275
	BISCUIT TORTONI	115
	TOTAL:	465
3 International	GREEK AVGOLEMONO SOUP	75
	CRUSTY LAMB CHOPS	400
	SPINACH SALAD WITH SUNFLOWER DRESSING	95
	BROILED PAPAYA	110
	TOTAL:	680
4 Golden Door Gourmet	MUSHROOM-STUFFED MUSHROOMS	80
	SOLE ALL'AGRO DI LIMONE	260
	ASPARAGUS MIMOSA	80
	STRAWBERRIES MYSTERY	95
	TOTAL:	515

5	VIRGIN MARY COCKTAIL WITH	
Quickie	CELERY	25
	CELERY ROOT AND APPLE SALAD	100
	FAST FONDUE WITH SKINNY DIPPERS	430
	PRUNE COMPOTE IN PORT	185
	TOTAL:	740

6	RADISHES ON ICE	55
Brunch or late,	CHIC CONSOMMÉ	45
late supper	SVELTE CHICKEN	205
	PEAS AU NATUREL	65
	CELESTIAL STRAWBERRY ANGEL CAKE	175
	TOTAL:	545

7	WHITE-WINE SPRITZER *(see page 225)*	45
Dinner for six	SMOKED SALMON SPEARS	55
	BROILED CHICKEN WITH MUSTARD	
	SAUCE	270
	GLAZED NEW POTATOES	90
	MEDITERRANEAN TOMATO SALAD	65
	SIMPLY CHEESECAKE	175
	TOTAL:	700

VERY LOW CAL

BROILED SHRIMP

(Each serving, 210 calories)

6 very large (about 5 inches long) raw, unpeeled shrimp or about ⅔ pound largest size
2 tablespoons 100% corn-oil margarine

1 tablespoon lemon juice
1 tablespoon white wine, dry vermouth, or water

Prepare shrimp to be broiled in shells with tails intact this way: Slit each shrimp lengthwise through shell down vein just far enough to butterfly (lay flat open); clean vein. Loosen meat within shell and score it lightly with knife blade in crisscross pattern to prevent curling. Lay each, shell side down, on foil-lined broiler pan. Preheat broiler.

Melt margarine in small saucepan. Brush about half on shrimp. Add lemon juice and wine to remaining margarine and heat (don't simmer).

Broil shrimp 6 inches from heat for about 5 minutes, or until very pink and beginning to brown (brush once with margarine-lemon mixture). Pour remaining hot mixture into small cups and serve as dipping sauce.

GREEN SALAD WITH ONION AND ORANGE
(Each serving, 90 calories)

1 clove garlic, halved
3 cups watercress sprigs or small pieces of curly endive or romaine (approximate)
2 thin slices sweet white or red onion, separated into rings, or 2 green onions, thinly sliced

1 small orange, peeled and thinly sliced
1 tablespoon corn oil or olive oil
1 teaspoon each red-wine vinegar and red wine (or water)
pinch of dry mustard
salt and pepper

Rub salad bowl with garlic. Add greens, onion, and orange. Blend remaining ingredients. Dribble over greens as you toss with fork. Add more vinegar, if needed.

PALACE MUHALLEBI
(Each serving, 130 calories)

The simple milk pudding Muhallebi is as popular in Turkey as fruit gelatin is in the United States.

4 teaspoons cornstarch
2 tablespoons sugar
¼ cup water
1 cup cold nonfat milk

5 whole cardamom pods, each slit on one side
several dashes of salt
1 tablespoon finely chopped toasted blanched almonds

In heavy saucepan mix cornstarch with sugar and stir in water; add milk, cardamom, and salt. Cook over very low heat for about 10 minutes, stirring often (do not simmer). When pudding begins to thicken, stir constantly until thick. Remove from heat and discard cardamom.

Pour into sherbet or parfait glasses and cover with wax paper to prevent skin from forming. Serve warm, chilled, or the Turkish way— at room temperature with almonds on top.

VEGETARIAN

WATER CHESTNUTS RUMAKI

(Each serving, 75 calories)

16 whole canned water chestnuts, well drained
1 tablespoon soy sauce

¼ teaspoon grated fresh ginger root, or several dashes ground ginger
2 teaspoons sugar

Marinate chestnuts in soy sauce and ginger for at least 10 minutes. Drain well in strainer. Preheat oven to 450° F. or preheat broiler.

Put chestnuts on plate and sprinkle with sugar, rolling each chestnut to coat thoroughly. Spear each with a pick (for broiling, spear at sides so picks do not stick upward and burn).

Bake on a foil-lined pan for about 5 minutes, or until hot and glazed. Or broil 4 inches from heat for about 2 minutes, turn, and broil a minute or so more until glazed.

FRESH FRUIT PLATE WITH PEACH DRESSING

(Each serving, 275 calories)

1 small head butter lettuce, or other soft lettuce
2 large fresh peaches, peeled, halved, and pitted
1 cup low-fat yogurt
½ cup low-fat cottage cheese
1 medium-sized grapefruit, peeled and divided into 6 wedges

½ medium-sized cantaloupe, peeled and cut into 6 wedges
10 large strawberries
1 bunch watercress
ground nutmeg
2 mint sprigs (optional)

For each serving, make a bed of the outside lettuce leaves on a dinner plate. Coarsely shred remaining lettuce. Place a small custard cup or Oriental teacup in center of plate. Heap shredded lettuce into and over it. Place 1 peach half, pitted side up, on top of each cup.

For dressing, combine yogurt and remaining 2 peach halves in blender and purée. Chill.

Form cottage cheese into 2 balls. Place on each peach half. Around side of each plate, arrange 3 grapefruit wedges, 3 cantaloupe wedges, and 5 strawberries. Fill spaces between fruit groups with watercress.

Pour dressing over peach mound. Sprinkle liberally with nutmeg and add a mint sprig on top.

BISCUIT TORTONI

(Each serving, 115 calories)

Our version retains the original flavor of the classic dessert and tastes surprisingly rich. Another surprise: it takes only 5 minutes to prepare for freezing.

1/4 cup each nonfat dry-milk powder and ice-cold water
2 teaspoons fresh lemon juice
5 teaspoons sugar
1 teaspoon sherry
1/4 teaspoon vanilla extract
1/8 teaspoon almond extract
1 tablespoon slivered blanched almonds, toasted

Combine milk powder and water in mixing bowl. Beat with an electric mixer until mixture resembles softly whipped cream. Continue to beat while sprinkling in lemon juice, sugar, sherry, vanilla extract, and almond extract. Beat until smooth and creamy like a light meringue. Heap into chilled custard cups or large paper baking cups in a chilled muffin pan. Put in freezer while preparing nuts.

Whirl almonds in blender to grind (or chop as finely as possible). Sprinkle over desserts to cover tops completely. Tortoni may be eaten partially frozen, or fully frozen (it takes about 1 hour). However, freezing more than about 1½ hours may produce ice crystals which spoil the smooth texture.

GREEK AVGOLEMONO SOUP
(Each serving, 75 calories)

1 egg
1½ tablespoons fresh lemon juice
2 cups chicken broth (see page 278)

grated lemon peel, minced parsley, or fresh mint for garnish

In a bowl, blend egg and lemon juice. Heat broth until boiling, then remove from heat. Beat a small amount of the hot broth into the eggs, then add to remaining broth, beating constantly. Heat through, continuing to stir constantly. Serve hot. Sprinkle one or more of the garnishes on top.

CRUSTY LAMB CHOPS
(Each serving of two chops, 400 calories)

2 tablespoons nonfat milk
1 tablespoon whole-wheat flour
2 tablespoons plain toasted wheat germ
2 teaspoons polyunsaturated oil

4 loin lamb chops (5 ounces each before trimming), trimmed of all fat, at room temperature
salt and pepper

Put milk in bowl. On a plate, blend flour and wheat germ. Pour 1 teaspoon oil in small frying pan over medium heat and turn pan to distribute evenly.

Dip each chop in milk, then coat in flour-wheat germ mixture, which has been seasoned with salt and pepper. Broil about 5 minutes, or until brown and crusty. Turn, adding the remaining 1 teaspoon oil. Broil about 5 minutes more, or until done to your liking.

SPINACH SALAD WITH SUNFLOWER DRESSING
(Each serving, 95 calories)

4 cups torn fresh spinach leaves (or whole small inside leaves, for a more elegant salad)
2 tablespoons olive oil

1 tablespoon lemon juice
tarragon and nutmeg
lemon (for grated peel)
2 tablespoons sunflower seeds

Put greens in bowl. Mix oil, lemon juice, several pinches of pulverized tarragon, and a dash of nutmeg. Grate a tiny bit of lemon peel onto greens. Dribble on dressing and toss with fork. Divide into two salad bowls. Sprinkle sunflower seeds on top.

BROILED PAPAYA
(Each serving, 110 calories)

1 ripe but firm papaya
 (about 8 ounces)
1 tablespoon lemon or lime juice

2 teaspoons dark brown sugar
2 tablespoons shredded coconut
lemon or lime wedges

Cut papaya in half lengthwise and discard seeds. Cut 8 slashes around sides (into fruit, but not through to the skin). Sprinkle juice over tops and into cavities. Sprinkle with sugar.

Preheat broiler. Broil fruit 6 inches from heat for about 5 minutes, or until very hot. Sprinkle coconut into cavities and broil again for about 1 or 2 minutes, or just until coconut is toasted. Watch carefully —coconut can burn quickly. Serve hot with lemon wedges.

GOLDEN DOOR GOURMET
MUSHROOM-STUFFED MUSHROOMS
(Each serving, 80 calories)

6 large mushrooms
 (at least 2 inches wide)
1 thin slice onion, chopped
2 teaspoons 100% corn-oil
 margarine

2 tablespoons dry vermouth or
 water
salt and pepper
¼ teaspoon each basil and
 oregano

Remove mushroom stems and chop. In a saucepan sauté stems and onion in margarine until they begin to brown. Spoon into mushroom caps and return to pan. Pour in vermouth. Sprinkle seasonings on caps.

Cover and simmer for about 10 minutes, or until about 1 tablespoon liquid remains. Serve hot with liquid spooned over.

SOLE ALL'AGRO DI LIMONE
(Each serving, 260 calories)

⅔ pound fillet of sole or other mild white fish (preferably 2 pieces of equal size)

salt and pepper

1 tablespoon unbleached flour

2 teaspoons corn or olive oil

1 tablespoon 100% corn-oil margarine

1½ teaspoons lemon juice

¼ cup dry white wine or dry vermouth

1 tablespoon minced parsley

4 thin lemon slices

paprika

Sprinkle the fish with salt and pepper and lightly coat with flour. In a small frying pan, heat the oil over medium-high heat. Sprinkle 1 teaspoon flour over oil and add fish. Cook about 2 minutes, then turn.

Cut margarine into 6 tiny pieces and add at intervals around sides of pan. Blend lemon juice and wine. Pour around sides of pan and dribble over fish. Simmer gently, uncovered, until liquid is slightly thickened and reduced. Total cooking time should be no more than 5 or 6 minutes.

Transfer fish to warm plates. Add 2 teaspoons of the parsley to pan; stir, and spoon sauce over fish. Sprinkle 2 lemon slices with paprika, the other 2 with the remaining parsley, and decorate fish.

ASPARAGUS MIMOSA
(Each serving, 80 calories)

16 to 24 asparagus stalks (depending on size), trimmed and washed

2 teaspoons 100% corn-oil margarine

1 teaspoon lemon juice

½ hard-cooked egg, finely chopped

Steam asparagus over salted water until thick ends are barely tender but color is still brilliant green. Drain and arrange on platter. Dot with margarine, sprinkle with lemon juice, and arrange chopped egg down the center.

STRAWBERRIES MYSTERY
(Each serving, 95 calories)

16 large fresh strawberries
lime or lemon (for grated peel)
 2 sprigs fresh mint (optional)

Mystery Sauce Ingredients
¼ teaspoon almond extract
 1 teaspoon honey
¼ cup low-fat yogurt

dash of cinnamon
 1 teaspoon coffee powder
  (Turkish, espresso, instant, or
  ground coffee shaken through
  fine strainer)
 1 kiwi fruit, peeled, or 3 additional large strawberries

Cut stems off berries so they will sit flat, points up, in two shallow dishes.

Put sauce ingredients into blender in order listed and purée. Pour sauce over berries and garnish with additional fruit. Chill. Grate peel liberally over all; add mint.

QUICKIE
VIRGIN MARY COCKTAIL WITH CELERY
(Each serving, 25 calories)

A Bloody Mary cocktail without vodka is called a Virgin Mary.

1 cup tomato juice
½ teaspoon lemon juice
¼ teaspoon Worcestershire sauce,
  or more to taste

2 drops hot-pepper sauce, or
  more to taste
2 lemon slices
4 celery sticks

Blend juices and sauces. Fill glasses with ice, add lemon slices, and insert celery sticks. Pour in juice.

CELERY ROOT AND APPLE SALAD
(Each serving, 100 calories)

Served on crisp butter lettuce, this makes an excellent winter salad. In the summer, substitute hearts of celery.

3 celery roots
juice of 1 lemon plus 1 tablespoon
   lemon juice
1 tablespoon mayonnaise
   (see page 276)
1 teaspoon Dijon mustard

¼ teaspoon freshly ground white
   pepper
1 Golden Delicious apple
2 tablespoons finely chopped
   parsley

Wash and peel the celery roots and then grate or chop finely. Sprinkle immediately with lemon juice to prevent discoloration. In a bowl combine the mayonnaise, mustard, 1 tablespoon lemon juice, and pepper and stir with a wire whisk to blend thoroughly. Add dressing to the grated celery. Grate apple and add to salad. Mix together and serve on a bed of lettuce. Sprinkle generously with chopped parsley.

FAST FONDUE WITH SKINNY DIPPERS

(Each serving, 280 calories for fondue, 150 calories for dippers)

½ clove garlic, cut in pieces
½ cup cold water
2 tablespoons cornstarch
½ cup dry white wine or dry
   vermouth
¼ pound Swiss, Gruyère, or
   Monterey Jack cheese,
   shredded
⅛ teaspoon salt

pepper (preferably white)
½ teaspoon dry mustard

For Dipping:
raw cauliflowerettes
raw mushrooms
raw zucchini sticks
raw broccoli flowerettes
4 Italian bread sticks

Rub a fondue pot or heavy saucepan with garlic. Mix 1 tablespoon or more of the water with cornstarch to make a smooth paste; set aside. Combine wine and remaining water in fondue pot and cook over moderately high heat until liquid is almost boiling. Gradually add cheese, stirring constantly until cheese melts; *do not boil.* Add cornstarch mixture. Continue cooking until fondue begins to thicken. Season with salt, pepper, and mustard. If mixture is not cooked in a fondue pot, transfer to a container that can be placed over a candlewarmer or other heating device at the table. Dip vegetables and bread sticks in fondue to eat. *California Fondue Variation:* Use Monterey Jack cheese. Season with crushed dried red chiles or chopped green chiles, either the mild type or fiery *jalapeños*.

PRUNE COMPOTE IN PORT
(Each serving, 185 calories)

In the summer, make this dish with fresh plums.

10 medium-sized prunes
½ cup port (any type)
¼ cup water

2 thin slices lemon
1 cinnamon stick, broken in half
6 whole cloves

Combine all the ingredients in a saucepan, cover, and simmer for about 15 minutes, or until prunes are tender. Serve cold, cool, or warm (with liquid). Divide lemon slices and spices between the two bowls. *Fresh Plum Variation:* Use 6 firm purple or red plums. Cut a slit in each so the skin will split attractively. Simmer in the poaching mixture for about 5 minutes, just until plums begin to soften. (Plums contain 5 additional calories per serving.)

BRUNCH OR LATE, LATE SUPPER
RADISHES ON ICE
(Each serving, 55 calories)

12 red radishes with leaves
1 tray ice, cracked or crushed

1 ounce caviar (sturgeon or lumpfish)

Trim off all but the small inside radish leaves and cut off roots. Fill wide bowl or platter with ice. "Replant" radishes in ice. Fill small dish with caviar and center in the ice. Dip radishes into caviar.

CHIC CONSOMMÉ
(Each serving, 45 calories)

2 cups homemade consommé or chicken broth (see recipe page 278)
2 teaspoons sherry

2 small bay leaves or 6 very thin slices raw ginger
4 whole black peppercorns

Combine all the ingredients and heat through. Serve in wide soup bowls with garnishing spices divided equally.
Note: Add spices just before heating and serving so that flavor does not get too strong.

SVELTE CHICKEN
(Each serving, 205 calories)

1 tablespoon corn oil or olive oil
1 chicken breast, halved and skinless
salt, pepper, and paprika
½ teaspoon each oregano and summer savory (optional) or 1

teaspoon dried rosemary leaves (or 4 long sprigs fresh rosemary)
2 thin slices lemon
2 small bay leaves

Spread half the oil on the bottom of a small baking pan. Place chicken in pan and brush remaining oil on top.

Sprinkle with salt, pepper, and paprika to color delicately; then add oregano and savory. Lay a lemon slice on each breast and tuck a bay leaf at the side. (Or lay fresh rosemary on, then lemon, and omit bay leaves.)

Bake, uncovered, at 350° F. for about 40 minutes, or until delicate brown but still moist-looking. Serve hot or at room temperature with lemon and herbs still in place.

PEAS AU NATUREL
(Each serving, 65 calories)

½ pound Chinese pea pods or very young peas in pods
¾ cup water

⅛ teaspoon salt
½ teaspoon 100% corn-oil margarine

In a small saucepan, combine the whole unshelled pea pods, water, and salt. Cover and simmer about 10 to 15 minutes for green peas; 2 minutes for pea pods. Test a pod with large peas to see if they are soft.

Meanwhile, divide the margarine into 2 small cups on two plates. Drain peas and pile on plates. Pour liquid into cups. Eat pod and all.

CELESTIAL STRAWBERRY ANGEL CAKE
(Each serving, 175 calories)

2 slices angel food cake, each slice 1/12 of an 8-inch cake

3/4 cup thinly sliced or crushed strawberries

1/3 cup low-fat yogurt

2 teaspoons brown sugar or kirsch

Garnish: 2 whole strawberries and 2 mint sprigs (optional)

Put each slice of cake in a bowl. Add 2 tablespoons sliced berries to yogurt and spoon rest on cake.

Blend sugar into yogurt, stirring until berries color sauce. Pour over cake. Decorate each with whole berry and a mint sprig. Serve immediately or chill.

DINNER FOR SIX
SMOKED SALMON SPEARS
(Each serving, 55 calories)

6 ounces Nova Scotia or Scotch smoked salmon

12 cucumber spears

freshly ground black pepper

lemon wedges

Cut salmon into 12 lengthwise strips. Wrap each around a cucumber spear. Guests can sprinkle on freshly ground black pepper and lemon juice to taste.

BROILED CHICKEN WITH MUSTARD SAUCE
(Each serving, 270 calories)

6 chicken-breast halves

3 tablespoons 100% corn-oil margarine, melted

1 tablespoon unbleached flour

1 tablespoon dry mustard

1 1/2 teaspoons fresh or 1/2 teaspoon dried dill, minced

1/4 teaspoon white pepper

1/4 teaspoon salt

3/4 cup low-fat milk

4 egg yolks, beaten

3 tablespoons lemon juice

Preheat broiler. Place skinless breasts on a rack 5 inches from heat. Brush with half the margarine. Broil for 15 minutes. Turn, brush with remaining margarine and broil another 15 minutes, or until done.

While the chicken is broiling, combine flour, mustard, dill, salt, and pepper in top of double boiler. Combine milk and yolks and stir in. Place over boiling water. Cook, stirring constantly, until mixture thickens. Stir in lemon juice. Spoon sauce over the broiled chicken breasts or other broiled foods such as fish.

GLAZED NEW POTATOES
(Each serving, 90 calories)

6 new potatoes about 3 inches long (white or red-skinned type) or about 1½ pounds tiny new potatoes

1 tablespoon 100% corn-oil margarine
1 teaspoon honey

Cook unpeeled potatoes in salted water until tender; drain and keep hot. In a saucepan melt margarine, add potatoes, and turn to coat. Dribble in honey and turn just until coated and shiny.

MEDITERRANEAN TOMATO SALAD
(Each serving, 65 calories)

6 large romaine leaves
3 large fully ripe tomatoes, each cut into 4 slices
salt and pepper
6 parsley sprigs
6 lemon wedges

3 tablespoons minced fresh parsley
3 tablespoons chopped green onion
2 tablespoons olive oil

For each serving: Lay a romaine leaf on plate, top with 2 tomato slices, and season with salt and pepper. Tuck a parsley sprig at side and garnish with 1 lemon wedge.

Mix minced parsley with green onion. Sprinkle on tomatoes, then dribble oil on. Squeeze lemon on for tartness desired.

SIMPLY CHEESECAKE
(Each serving, 175 calories)

1½ teaspoons unflavored gelatin
¾ cup cold water
⅓ cup sugar
grated peel of 2 lemons
5 tablespoons fresh lemon juice

2 cups low-fat cottage cheese
1½ teaspoons each rum flavoring
and vanilla extract
¾ cup toasted granola or 18 to
24 whole strawberries

In a small saucepan, soften gelatin in water. Heat (but do not simmer), stirring until no gelatin granules are seen on spoon. Cool slightly; pour into blender with lemon peel and juice, cottage cheese, and flavorings. Whirl until lightly whipped. Pour into sherbet glasses. Or, if you want to unmold, use oiled tart pans or ½-cup molds. Chill until firm.

Whirl cereal in blender. At serving time, sprinkle crumbs on top of cheesecake or put 3 or 4 whole strawberries beside each serving.

□ DRESSINGS AND SAUCES

I present with pride The Golden Door's great, gourmet, low-calorie dressings and sauces. The key to The Golden Door's weight reduction with glorious eating is our collection of very special dressings and sauces which have been developed over the years. We use them to make fresh, simple, and quickly prepared basic foodstuffs even more tasty and elegant.

Use them when lunching and whenever you need dressings or sauces. You will find that we use them throughout the four weeks of dinner menus. The dressings and sauces are listed here alphabetically, according to the principal ingredient or generic term.

BUTTERMILK DRESSING
(Each tablespoon, 15 calories)

3 tablespoons polyunsaturated
oil
½ cup low-fat buttermilk
3 tablespoons vinegar
¼ cup catsup (see page 274)

¼ teaspoon dry English mustard
¼ teaspoon salt
⅓ cup peeled, seeded, and diced
cucumber

Place all the ingredients in a bowl and whisk until well blended. Makes 1 cup.

CATSUP

(Each tablespoon, 6 calories)

1 can whole tomatoes (28 ounces)
1 small onion, cut into chunks
1 carrot, cut into chunks
1 stalk celery, cut into chunks

6 large parsley sprigs, cut into pieces
2 teaspoons prepared white horseradish

Purée tomatoes in blender with juice, onion, carrot, celery, and parsley. Blend until smooth. Pour into a saucepan and boil rapidly, uncovered, for 15 minutes, stirring often, or until almost the desired consistency. Add horseradish and simmer, stirring constantly, until very thick, about 5 minutes longer. Makes 2½ cups.

TIPS: For a very smooth texture, you may blend fully cooked mixture again. Press through a coarse wire strainer to remove seeds and pulp.

For a more traditional catsup, season with 2 teaspoons vinegar and a bit of brown sugar or honey. Fresh tomatoes (2½ pounds) may be substituted if you want less salt. Peel tomatoes before blending by immersing in boiling water for 3 minutes, or until skin strips off easily.

Keep refrigerated. Use within 3 or 4 days. Or freeze small portions to use as needed.

CREAM SAUCE

(Each ½ cup, 80 calories)

2 cups instant nonfat milk
1 tablespoon 100% corn-oil margarine

2½ tablespoons unbleached flour
⅛ teaspoon salt

Bring milk to simmer in a saucepan. In another pan, melt the margarine and blend in the flour and salt, stirring constantly. Remove the flour-margarine mixture from the heat and slowly add the milk, stirring constantly with a wire whisk. Return the sauce to low heat and cook very slowly until mixture thickens. This makes about 2 cups thin cream sauce.

DILL DRESSING

(Each tablespoon, 12 calories)

1 teaspoon Dijon mustard
1 teaspoon Golden Door seasoning salt (see page 277)
1 teaspoon dried dill
1 clove garlic, minced

2 teaspoons chopped onion
2 teaspoons polyunsaturated oil
5 teaspoons wine vinegar
2 tablespoons water

Put mustard and all dry ingredients in a wooden salad bowl. Using a fork, crush everything together well. Add liquids and stir vigorously until well blended.

Serve on any greens with a slightly bitter taste: dandelion greens, endive, chicory, and the like. Makes ½ cup.

HOLLANDAISE

(Each ⅓ cup, 80 calories)

This is a rich, tangy mock hollandaise made without butter.

1 egg yolk
¼ cup nonfat milk
dash of nutmeg
dash of Golden Door seasoning
  salt (see page 277)

dash of white pepper
1 teaspoon lemon juice
½ cup plain low-fat yogurt

In the top of a double boiler, beat the egg yolk with a wire whisk until it turns light yellow. Still beating constantly, very slowly add the nonfat mik which has been blended with nutmeg, seasoning salt, and pepper. Place over boiling water and whisk for a minute before adding lemon juice.

When sauce has thickened, fold in yogurt and heat slightly. Makes ⅔ cup sauce.

LEMON DRESSING

(Each tablespoon, 30 calories)

½ cup polyunsaturated oil
¾ cup water
¾ cup fresh lemon juice
1 teaspoon Golden Door season-
    ing salt (see page 277)

½ cup low-fat yogurt
1 shallot, minced
1 clove garlic, minced

Place all ingredients in a blender and blend until smooth. Chill before using. Makes 2½ cups.

MAYONNAISE

(250 calories per recipe; 21 per tablespoon)

1 teaspoon fresh lemon juice
1 raw egg yolk
1 teaspoon Dijon mustard
2 small shallots, or 2 thin onion
    slices, or a mixture of the two,
    diced

pinch of salt and white pepper
2 hard-cooked egg yolks
½ cup low-fat yogurt

In a blender, combine the lemon juice, raw egg yolk, mustard, shallots, salt, and pepper. Blend until shallot is puréed. Crumble hard-cooked egg yolks into the container and blend again until creamy. If mix won't purée completely, add 1 or 2 tablespoons of yogurt. Fold egg mixture into yogurt (do not blend—mayonnaise will become too thin). Refrigerate. Will keep at least a week. Makes ¾ cup.

MUSTARD SAUCE

(Each tablespoon, 25 calories)

Excellent with broiled chicken, lamb, cold fish like salmon or tuna, or hot poached or broiled fish. Leftover sauce can be served with vegetables.

1 tablespoon unbleached flour
1 tablespoon dry mustard
1½ teaspoons fresh dill, minced,
    or ½ teaspoon dried dill weed
¼ teaspoon salt

¼ teaspoon white pepper
¾ cup skim milk
4 egg yolks, beaten
3 tablespoons lemon juice

In the top of a double boiler, combine flour, mustard, dill, salt, and pepper. Stir in milk and yolks. Place over boiling water and cook, stirring constantly, until mixture thickens. Stir in lemon juice. Serve hot. Makes 1 cup.

ORANGE DRESSING FOR FRUIT SALAD
(Each tablespoon, 20 calories)

2 tablespoons honey
1/4 cup fresh orange juice
1 egg
1/2 cup low-fat yogurt
pinch of nutmeg and salt

Place all ingredients in a blender and whirl until thoroughly mixed. Makes 1 cup.

GOLDEN DOOR SEASONING SALT

This "salt" seasons food beautifully and contributes its own original flavor to cooking.

3 ounces powdered vegetable broth
1/4 teaspoon garlic powder
1/8 teaspoon powdered thyme
1/4 teaspoon onion powder
1/4 teaspoon paprika
1/2 teaspoon powdered kelp
1/8 teaspoon ground celery seed
1/4 teaspoon white pepper
1/4 teaspoon dry mustard

Mix together and store in a closed container in a dry place.

THOUSAND ISLAND DRESSING
(Each tablespoon, 25 calories)

3 tablespoons tomato purée
3 tablespoons wine vinegar or fresh lemon juice
1 cup plain low-fat yogurt
1 teaspoon fresh horseradish
dash of hot-pepper sauce
3/4 cup chopped chives
3 whole pimientos, chopped
3 tablespoons polyunsaturated oil
1/2 cup water
salt to taste
1 hard-cooked egg, chopped

Place all the ingredients except egg in blender, and blend until well mixed. Pour dressing into a bowl and fold in chopped egg. Serve at once. Makes about 2 cups.

TIP: As a dip for raw vegetables, add some to plain yogurt.

TOMATO SAUCE

(Each ¼ cup, 40 calories)

Good over fish or ground-beef patties.

1 tablespoon polyunsaturated oil
1 clove garlic, finely chopped
¼ cup chopped onion
1 shallot, finely chopped
2 cups tomato purée
½ cup water
2 teaspoons fresh oregano, minced, or ¾ teaspoon dried oregano
3 leaves fresh basil, finely chopped, or ½ teaspoon crushed dried basil
2 bay leaves
2 teaspoons minced parsley
salt and pepper

Heat oil in large skillet and sauté garlic, onion, and shallot over medium heat until golden. Add tomato purée, water, and herbs and cook, uncovered, over low heat for 45 minutes, stirring occasionally to prevent sticking. Season with salt and pepper, if necessary. Makes 2 cups.

VEGETARIAN DRESSING DELIGHT

(Each tablespoon, 3 calories)

1 stalk celery, finely chopped
1 medium-sized tomato, peeled and quartered
¼ cup chopped chives
¼ cup chopped parsley
¼ cup chopped onion
1 cup water
4 tablespoons vinegar
2 teaspoons Golden Door seasoning salt (see page 277)

Place all ingredients in saucepan and bring to boil. Simmer for 5 minutes. Purée in blender. Chill before using. Makes 2 cups.

□ OUR BASIC BROTH

The classic chicken broth is a real help to fine cooking. Although canned or powdered bouillon may be used in a pinch, the home-prepared broth is infinitely better. Make it ahead when you have time and freeze it in small containers, ready for future use. A vegetarian should prepare a stock broth in a similar manner, but without meat.

CHICKEN BROTH

1 (3-pound) roasting chicken

5 carrots, peeled and cut in chunks

5 stalks celery

3 onions

5 cloves

5 peppercorns

1 teaspoon thyme

3 cloves garlic

parsley to taste

Place all the ingredients in a large pot with water to cover. Bring to a boil and then reduce heat to a slow simmer. Cook gently for 3 hours. Remove chicken from the pot, strip away the skin, and refrigerate chicken for use in other dishes. Boil broth rapidly for 30 minutes to reduce it. Strain through a sieve lined with cheesecloth. Chill broth and remove congealed fat from the surface before placing broth in storage containers. Freeze, if desired.

□ BREADS AND SPROUTS

OUR WONDERFUL WHOLE-WHEAT TECATE BREAD

(Makes 2 loaves—22 slices per loaf, 105 calories per slice)

2 packages yeast

4 cups warm water (105°–115° F. for dry yeast)

2 tablespoons honey

½ cup polyunsaturated oil

7½–8 cups stone-ground whole-wheat flour

Place yeast in a very large bowl. Add warm water and stir. Blend in honey and oil. While beating with an electric mixer, add flour gradually until dough pulls off the beaters cleanly. Turn dough out onto a floured board and knead until dough is no longer sticky. To knead, fold the dough toward you and push the outer edge of the dough down, toward you, and then away from you with the heel of your hand. The dough is ready when it is silky and feels slightly bouncy. The kneading will take about 8 to 10 minutes.

Place the dough in an oiled bowl, turning the dough once to oil the top. Cover with a clean cloth and allow to rise in a warm, draft-free spot until doubled in bulk, about 1 hour. (You can check to see if dough is ready by pressing the top with your finger. If a dent remains, the dough has risen enough.)

Punch the dough down; divide it in half and roll each half into a 12- x 15-inch oblong. Starting at the narrow end, roll up, jelly-roll fashion. Seal seam and fold over each end 1 inch. Place, seam side down, in a greased 9- x 5- x 3-inch bread pan. Cover and allow to rise again until doubled in bulk, about 1 hour.

Bake in a preheated 375° F. oven for 50 to 60 minutes, or until the loaf is well browned and has a hollow sound when rapped on top.

Cool bread on racks. To freeze, wrap in moisture- and vapor-proof wrapping paper, pressing out as much air as possible. May be stored, frozen, for about 4 months.

SPROUTS

Use sprouts in both fruit and vegetable salads, in sandwiches, as a garnish, and in homemade bread.

Wheat and many grains and seeds are at their best when sprouted. Nature's own growth processes modify the composition, which results in increased micronutrients, vitamins, and a more digestible protein. Wheat, alfalfa, and mung beans are most widely used for sprouting. However, it is fun to experiment, and soon you can have a year-round table garden in your kitchen.

Soak about a quarter of a cup of seeds overnight. In the morning, rinse in fresh water, drain, and place in an open-mouthed jar covered with cheesecloth or a bit of nylon net. Secure with a rubber band. Lay the jar at a 45° angle so that any surplus moisture will continue to drain. Rinse and drain every morning and evening with slightly warm water to keep the sprouts sweet. In three or four days reap the fruits of your labor. Sprouts can be kept for a day or two in the re- frigerator.

SPROUTED BREAKFAST BUNS

I begin every day with one of these buns. To me, they are the staff of life.

2 cups whole-wheat grains, sprout quality

¾ cup large black raisins

1 heaping tablespoon caraway seeds

Sprout as above 2 cups whole-wheat grains.

Using the finest blade on your electric or hand meat grinder, run the sprouts through twice (once if you have a Champion or similar multi-purpose juicer). Sprinkle over the ground sprouts the raisins and caraway seeds. Mix and form into small buns 3" in diameter and not over 1½" thick, or make a flat loaf of the same thickness.

Bake on a lightly oiled baking sheet at 350° for 50 minutes. Cool and store in refrigerator. Delicious served as is or toasted. Bake fresh buns every few days; as no yeast is used, the buns become very hard in a day or so.

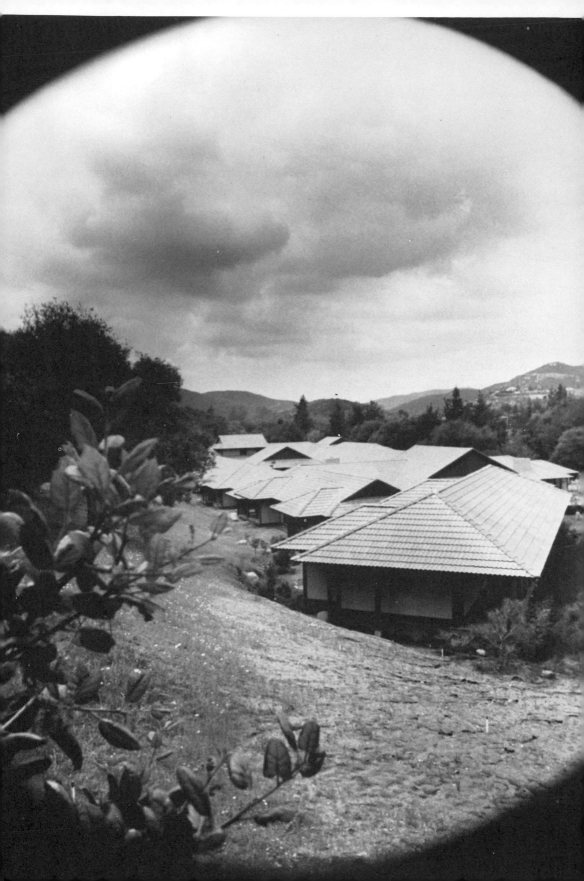

INDEX